Lorena Loor
Virginia Pincay

Biomass and health

Lorena Loor
Virginia Pincay

Biomass and health

Nursing interventions in patients with respiratory diseases associated with biomass smoke

ScienciaScripts

Imprint

Cover image: www.ingimage.com

This book is a translation from the original published under ISBN 978-613-9-43384-1.

Publisher:
Sciencia Scripts
is a trademark of
Dodo Books Indian Ocean Ltd. and OmniScriptum S.R.L publishing group

120 High Road, East Finchley, London, N2 9ED, United Kingdom
Str. Armeneasca 28/1, office 1, Chisinau MD-2012, Republic of Moldova, Europe
Printed at: see last page
ISBN: 978-620-8-12038-2

LIST OF CONTENTS

UNIVERSIDAD ESTATAL DEL SUR DE MANABÍ POSTGRADUATE INSTITUTE

MASTER'S DEGREE IN CARE MANAGEMENT

Title: Nursing interventions in patients with biomass smoke associated respiratory diseases

Author: Lcda Loor Alvarado Lorena María

Tutor: Lcda. Pincay Pin Virginia Esmeralda, Mg.

SUMMARY

Nursing interventions in patients with biomass smoke-associated respiratory diseases are essential to provide comprehensive care and promote improved respiratory health in these populations, focusing on assessment and monitoring, education and counselling, symptom management and treatment, promotion of treatment adherence, emotional support and stress management, and multidisciplinary care coordination, aimed at improving patient education for prevention. The main **objective** of this research was to apply nursing interventions through the promotion and prevention of respiratory diseases associated with biomass smoke. For this purpose, a descriptive and observational **methodology** was applied, with a quantitative, non-experimental and longitudinal approach. The **results** obtained suggest that before the nursing interventions, knowledge about the dangers of biomass smoke in patients was null, however, after the application of the talks given to the users and the development of the educational guide, the understanding of the participants increased to a great extent. It was **concluded** that nursing activities focused on the promotion and prevention of respiratory diseases associated with biomass smoke were essential for education and multidisciplinary collaboration, the development of the educational guide influences behavioural change towards healthier and safer practices in relation to exposure to biomass smoke by understanding the negative health effects.

Keywords: respiratory disorders, biomass, wood, nursing staff.

2. CONTENT OF THE REPORT

2.1 Introduction of the degree project

Respiratory diseases affect the lungs directly and can arise from pulmonary, cardiovascular, emotional and severe life-threatening causes, some diseases such as chronic obstructive pulmonary disease (COPD), asthma, bronchiolitis are due to major risk factors associated with smoking, indoor and outdoor air pollution, occupational exposures and poverty(1).

This research work is focused on nursing interventions for patients with respiratory diseases associated with the inhalation of biomass smoke, which is caused by constant exposure to smoke particles from biofuels, causing health problems for the world's population, The highest incidence of respiratory diseases is caused by smoke from wood, coal and tobacco, as the most harmful organic compounds are found inside homes due to the use of wood-burning cookers, affecting children and the elderly, the most vulnerable age group(2).

People who are exposed to biomass smoke on a regular basis, such as those living in rural areas where it is common to cook and heat with this fuel are not aware of this issue and the minimal risk of an allergy triggered by this material, to the increased risk of developing respiratory complications and diseases such as chronic bronchitis, asthma and COPD, has also been linked to an increased risk of lung cancer.

According to the World Health Organisation (WHO), exposure to household air pollution (HAP) from burning biomass fuels for cooking and heating is a major public health problem, particularly in low- and middle-income countries. It is estimated that HAP is responsible for approximately 4 million deaths per year, mainly due to respiratory diseases such as pneumonia and chronic obstructive pulmonary disease (COPD), the smoke produced by these fuels contains a complex mixture of harmful pollutants, including fine particulate matter (PM), carbon monoxide (CO) and polycyclic aromatic hydrocarbons (PAHs)(3).

"According to studies conducted according to the WHO in 2018, household air pollution causes non-communicable diseases that can start with acute respiratory diseases and go up to chronic diseases, cardiovascular diseases, strokes, chronic obstructive pulmonary disease (COPD), lung cancer, complications caused by toxic biomass smoke material" (4).

In Latin America according to the World Health Organisation (WHO) it has been estimated that exposure to domestic air pollution from burning biomass fuels is responsible for approximately 40,000 deaths per year, children and pregnant women are especially vulnerable to the harmful effects of biomass smoke, which can have long-term effects on respiratory health and development (5).

In Ecuador there is a population of 2,680 people affected by acute respiratory diseases, of which 1,395 are women and 1,285 are men, with the highest number of cases occurring in the provinces of Pichincha and Guayas (6). This incidence has a high recurrence rate, occurring between 4 to 6 times per year in urban areas and 5 to 8 times in rural areas. The fact of living in rural communities in the Manabí area indicates that accessibility to a health centre for treatment is more difficult, especially for those living in more remote areas (7).

Nursing interventions play a vital role in the prevention and management of respiratory diseases associated with biomass smoke. Nurses can provide education to patients and their families, assess and monitor symptoms, administer medications and provide respiratory care to improve patient outcomes.

Several studies have highlighted the importance of nursing interventions in the management of respiratory diseases associated with biomass smoke, with several studies finding that interventions aimed at reducing exposure to biomass smoke can be effective in improving respiratory health outcomes. Other authors emphasised the importance of a multidisciplinary approach to the management of respiratory diseases associated with biomass smoke, with nurses playing a crucial role in patient education and self-care support (8).

Nursing interventions are critical in the prevention and management of respiratory diseases associated with biomass smoke exposure. Through education, assessment, monitoring, medication administration and respiratory care, nurses can help improve patient outcomes and reduce the burden of these diseases.

During this time approximately 100 patients over 18 years of age with respiratory disorders were studied and attended in the Noboa parish, of which 30 cases were selected by means of a non-probabilistic sampling by convenience, it is necessary to highlight that this problem arises due to the increase in the use of firewood as fuel for cooking and burning rubbish, In order to solve this problem, the thesis project seeks to improve the health of residents by implementing nursing interventions and continuing education on the damage caused by exposure to biomass smoke on individual health.

2.2 Statement of the research problem

Nowadays, there is frequent exposure to biomass smoke from the burning of different elements, such as crop residues, constant smoking, burning of rubbish in the sector, use of firewood in the kitchen, factors that cause serious health risks for the individual, the family and the community, as well as the constant passage of motorised vehicles that increase the biomass through the smoke emanating from the engines.

Respiratory diseases related to exposure to biomass smoke is a major public health problem in many parts of the world, especially in rural areas and developing countries. Globally, according to WHO data, more than 3.8 million individuals die from respiratory diseases attributed to biomass smoke and organic matter as cooking fuel, statistically 27% of these deaths are due to childhood and adult pneumonia, 20% COPD and 8% lung cancer (9).

Currently, several developing countries in Latin America and the Caribbean are experiencing accelerated growth and rapid urbanisation, with rates reaching around 80%, respectively coal/biomass fuel consumption is only 16%, there are still many countries and rural areas that rely heavily on biomass fuel (10). In Central American regions, more than 90 % of rural households and about half of urban households continue to rely on biomass for cooking and cookers, adding to the burden of indoor pollutants (11).

According to INEC statistics in Ecuador, 11% of households in urban areas and 77% of households in rural areas use wood as fuel for cooking and heating their homes. The use of wood as fuel is a common practice, especially in rural areas of developing countries, but has also been observed in developed countries in recent decades (12).

In Noboa parish, the increased use of wood as fuel for cooking and rubbish burning has resulted in high levels of smoke emissions, negatively affecting the respiratory health of residents, and despite efforts to reduce smoke exposure, there has been limited success in mitigating health impacts, Lack of knowledge and awareness of the risks of exposure to biomass smoke among residents is also a major problem, the community does not have the necessary information to prevent the dangers of contracting respiratory diseases, due to the deficit of nursing intervention due to lack of education, these diseases can become chronic.

Due to all these factors that are present in this community, there was a need to carry out this research project in order to improve the current situation.

2.3 Problem formulation

Against this background, the following question arises:

How does inadequate nursing intervention affect patients with respiratory diseases associated with biomass smoke?

2.4 Definition of the object of research

Nursing intervention.

2.5 General objective

Apply nursing interventions in patients with respiratory diseases associated with biomass smoke.

2.6 Specific objectives

- To determine the level of knowledge of users about respiratory diseases associated with biomass smoke.
- Describe nursing activities through the promotion and prevention of respiratory diseases associated with biomass smoke.
- Define the main health determinants influencing respiratory diseases associated with biomass smoke.
- Design an education guide on respiratory diseases associated with biomass smoke.

2.7 Field of action or study

Nursing interventions in patients with respiratory diseases.

2.8 Hypothetical assumptions

The effectiveness of nursing interventions through the promotion and prevention of respiratory diseases associated with biomass smoke will decrease the complications of respiratory diseases and improve quality of life. The **independent variable** is defined as nursing interventions and the **dependent variable** as respiratory diseases associated with biomass smoke.

2.8.1. Research task

- To address and fulfil the first objective, two surveys were administered to the study population to assess patients' knowledge of biomass smoke and how harmful it is to their health, the questions determined the importance of having a basis on the subject and to compare the degree of existing knowledge.
- To meet this objective, users were asked whether nursing staff carried out activities to prevent the risk of respiratory diseases associated with biomass smoke, which provided evidence-based recommendations and best practices for nurses to follow, promoting a standardised and multidisciplinary approach to patient care.
- To address and fulfil the third objective, a survey was carried out among the nursing staff of the Noboa Health Centre where the objective of the study was addressed, identifying the main health determinants that contribute to the progression of these diseases.
- The fourth objective was met through the development of the educational guide which is aimed at affected patients, crucial to promote standardised care, prevent disease progression, provide effective care and encourage a multidisciplinary approach to patient care.

2.9 Justification

Nursing interventions are designed to address the specific needs of individual patients, often tailored to the patient's age, health status, cultural background, personal preferences, a variety of skills, techniques are used to implement these interventions, including assessment, communication, critical thinking, problem solving, effective nursing interventions can help improve patient outcomes, reduce complications, hospital readmissions and promote overall health and well-being.

According to the National Institute of Public Health, there are a total of 86,531 deaths attributed to the domestic use of solid fuels produced by the inhalation of biomass smoke. This is due to the lack of knowledge about the factors that can lead to respiratory disease, which is why the individual does not take the correct preventive measures to avoid these diseases (13).

This work is carried out with the purpose of providing information for the knowledge of the most common respiratory diseases produced by the inhalation of biomass smoke, it also tries to detail the main factor that causes it in the parish Noboa, education on the burning of biomass will serve to people, families and communities to improve their lifestyle, both the nursing staff for further research and preventive actions that promote through education.

The following research is feasible because it has the authorisation of the district health director 13D04 24 de Mayo - Santa Ana - Olmedo. This study is feasible because it has human, economic, technological and bibliographic resources, which demonstrate the importance of the subject, as well as a survey to obtain accurate results and collect all the necessary and indispensable data for the research.

The aim of this research is to apply nursing interventions in patients with respiratory diseases associated with biomass smoke through promotion and prevention that benefits patients, families and communities in the Noboa parish by receiving timely information necessary to reduce the risk of falling ill or complicating respiratory diseases caused by biomass smoke, a factor that negatively affects the health of those exposed and to produce positive changes through the different educational strategies applied by the researcher as the indirect beneficiary.

2.10 Methodology and methods

Type of study: This is a descriptive, observational research with a quantitative design.

Descriptive: because it focuses on describing nursing interventions in patients with respiratory diseases associated with biomass smoke in a specific geographical area and during a specific period of time (April-June 2023).

Observational: focuses on observing the nursing interventions in these patients, additionally observing and recording what happens in the population without manipulating any variable or treatment.

Study design: It has a quantitative, non-experimental, longitudinal approach.

Quantitative: involves the collection of numerical data through the measurement of quantitative variables, with the aim of establishing causal relationships between variables.

Non-experimental: review of medical records, nursing records of patients, direct observation of patients and collection of demographic data.

Longitudinal: involves the selection of a group of patients, who are assessed at different points in time to measure the evolution of their knowledge.

Population: 100 patients treated for respiratory diseases at the Noboa Parish Health Centre.

Sample: The sample consisted of 30 patients diagnosed with respiratory diseases associated with biomass smoke, who were selected by non-probabilistic convenience sampling and through medical care verified in the PRAS system.

Inclusion criteria

- Patients diagnosed with respiratory diseases associated with biomass smoke.
- Patients who voluntarily participate in the research and sign the informed consent form.

Exclusion criteria

- People who do not wish to participate in the research study.
- People with respiratory diseases associated with other factors.

Computer tools and statistical packages used for the processing and analysis of the data obtained.

A bibliographic and documentary review was carried out on the subject in different medical databases and official pages of organisations such as: pubmed, Elsevier, academic Google, books and reports.

For the collection of the first data, Microsoft Word and Excel 2020 programmes were used, and the processing was carried out with a statistical programme (SPSS), which provides relevant information to support the research, objectives and results obtained.

Procedure: The study is based on determining how the use of biomass in the parish of Noboa influences daily practice, due to this factor that negatively affects the health of the inhabitants because of the lack of knowledge that exists in the parish. In order to meet the objectives set out, a descriptive, observational study of quantitative design and longitudinal cohort was used, through the application of surveys aimed at patients with respiratory diseases due to the use of biomass, a factor that influences the object of this research, in addition to a nursing education guide that helps to improve lifestyle and knowledge about the use of biomass.

Ethical considerations

Equitable subject selection: Equitable subject selection requires that science, not vulnerability or social stigma, powerlessness or factors unrelated to the purpose of the research, dictate who is included as a likely subject.

Informed consent: The purpose of informed consent is to ensure that individuals participate in proposed research only when it is compatible with their values, interests and preferences; and that they do so of their own free will with sufficient knowledge to decide responsibly about themselves.

Justice: All nurses at the Noboa Health Centre have the same probability of participating in the study and those who meet the inclusion criteria will be selected.

2.11 Research methods

In order to reach the results of this study, empirical and statistical methods were applied, such as:

Surveys: structured questionnaires to collect information on the frequency of respiratory symptoms and other relevant variables.

Interview: The interview was used as it is a way of collecting data for the research, which makes it a useful strategy for the project.

Medical records: patient data that can be collected from electronic medical records, such as the PRAS system.

Literature review: the elaboration of the state of the art will require related research, theories and statistical data from articles and systematic explorations.

3. CHAPTER 1. THEORETICAL BACKGROUND

3.1 Theoretical framework of reference Nursing interventions

Nurses play a key role in the health care system and are central to providing high quality health care services. It is crucial that the skills and competencies of nurses are compatible with the demands of the health service. Competence has been defined as a combination of knowledge, skills, attitudes and assessments, and has also been described as the professional ability to effectively use a combination of knowledge, skills, personal qualities and understanding not only in predictable specialised situations, but also in unexpected and unstable circumstances (14).

The global prevalence of respiratory diseases and problems is increasing, so research into new treatment and prevention techniques is essential.

In addition, a rescue strategy has been implemented to treat acute respiratory distress syndrome by prone ventilation of critically ill patients, although this technique may have negative side effects, such as skin damage(15).

Orem's model of self-care

Nursing's distinctive knowledge is applied within an increasingly complex world of interprofessional and interdisciplinary practice. With the explosion of knowledge in basic science, technology and other health care disciplines, nursing's future theoretical contributions must include concepts and outcomes fully understood and valued by all members of the health care team (16).

Self-care

The World Health Organisation defines self-care as "the ability of individuals, families and communities to promote health, prevent disease, maintain health and cope with illness and disability with or without the support of a health care system provider" (Walker, 2020).

Recently, El-Ostra described an acceleration of interest in general self-care primarily to address increased health care costs and the demands of health and social systems, his review of academic and lay literature revealed 32 models, theories and frameworks of self-care, and international collaboration on mid-range self-care theories specific to chronic illness has impressive applications for nursing practice and research (18).

People-centred care

The global people-centred initiative provides a framework for empowering and engaging people in their health care to improve health and well-being, elements of the global people-centred movement, such as empowering people through education and self-care, are congruent with the strengths of Orem's SCDNT and provide evidence of its relevance now and in the next decade (19).

Orem's model in patients with respiratory diseases

Orem's nursing model, also known as nursing self-care theory, can be applied to patients with respiratory problems. This model emphasises the patient's ability to participate in their own care and the nurse's role in assisting them to achieve self-care (20).

According to Orem's model, nursing interventions for patients with respiratory problems should focus on three areas.

Self-care requirements

These are the actions patients must take to maintain or improve their respiratory function. Nursing interventions may include teaching patients proper breathing techniques, the use of medications such as bronchodilators or inhalers, and the importance of avoiding triggers that may exacerbate their respiratory symptoms(21).

Self-care deficits

These are the areas where patients need assistance in performing self-care activities related to their respiratory problems. Nursing interventions may include providing assistance with activities of daily living, such as bathing or dressing, and monitoring vital signs, such as oxygen saturation levels (21).

Self-care education

It involves providing patients with the knowledge and skills necessary to perform self-care activities related to their respiratory problems. Nursing interventions may include teaching patients about proper nutrition, exercise and the use of equipment such as oxygen tanks or nebulisers (21).

Respiratory system

The respiratory system is mainly made up of several parts, including the nose, oropharynx, larynx, trachea, bronchi, bronchioles and lungs, which in turn are divided into individual lobes and more than 300 million alveoli, the latter being essential for gas exchange, contraction of the primary muscle of respiration, the diaphragm, is controlled by the nerve roots of C3, C4 and C5, which innervate it via the phrenic nerve, while inspiratory muscles, such as the external intercostal muscles, are used more during physical exercise and in situations of respiratory distress (22).

Respiratory diseases

The lungs also perform a variety of non-respiratory functions, such as protection against infectious agents, elimination of waste products, and production of hormones and other chemicals important to the body. Respiratory diseases can have a variety of causes, including exposure to toxic substances, accidents and harmful habits such as smoking. Genetic factors and any condition that affects lung development can also contribute to these diseases (23).

Chronic respiratory diseases (CRDs) are common worldwide and are mainly due to harmful environmental, occupational and behavioural inhalation exposures (24). These diseases include chronic obstructive pulmonary disease (COPD), asthma, interstitial lung diseases, pulmonary sarcoidosis and pneumoconiosis, such as silicosis and asbestosis, yet despite their prevalence, CRDs have received less attention and research funding compared to other diseases, such as cardiovascular disease, cancer, stroke, diabetes mellitus and Alzheimer's disease (25).

Risk factors

It is important to mention that there are several factors that can induce the presence or appearance of an infection in the respiratory system, however, prevention is the best measure that can be taken for this worldwide problem (26).

Risk factors are characteristics that can influence the likelihood that a person will experience negative events; in the case of respiratory diseases, they are considered risk factors:

- Tobacco and alcohol use.
- Environmental pollutants (burning of crop residues, solid and organic waste).
- General lifestyle of a person (presence of domestic animals in the household and hygiene within the household).

Environmental exposures: Exposure to air pollution, second-hand smoke, dust and occupational chemicals and other environmental pollutants can increase the risk of respiratory diseases such as asthma, chronic obstructive pulmonary disease (COPD) and lung cancer (27).

Lifestyle choices: tobacco smoking, vaping and exposure to e-cigarette aerosols can lead to respiratory diseases such as lung cancer, COPD and respiratory infections (27)'.

Genetic predispositions: certain genetic variants have been associated with increased susceptibility to respiratory diseases such as asthma, cystic fibrosis and pulmonary fibrosis (27).

Underlying health conditions: Chronic diseases such as heart disease, diabetes and obesity have been linked to an increased risk of respiratory diseases such as COPD and pneumonia (28).

Biomass smoke

Biomass smoke is the smoke produced by burning organic material, such as wood, charcoal, crop residues and animal waste, and is a major source of air pollution, especially in rural areas where biomass is commonly used for cooking and heating.

Studies have shown that biomass smoke contains a complex mixture of gases and particles, including carbon monoxide, nitrogen oxides, volatile organic compounds and particulate matter. These pollutants can have a wide range of adverse health effects, including respiratory problems, cardiovascular disease and cancer (29).

Although biomass fuel is mostly used by women in developing countries for cooking in the home, it is also used in developed countries as the main source of heating by about 5% of households in Australia through the use of wood-burning cookers, although incomplete combustion of biomass fuels (BMF) in cooking and heating results mainly idomestic air pollution (HAP), it also contributes significantly tambient (outdoor) air pollution (AAP), and accounts for approximately 10-30% of ambient fine particulate matter (30).

Components

The exact chemical composition of biomass smoke depends on fuel type, combustion temperature, whether an open fire or a free radical incinerator is used and local conditions, air pollution components are mixtures of solid, liquid and mixed particles suspended in the air, common PM components include nitrates, sulphates, PAHs, endotoxins and metals such as iron, copper, nickel, zinc and vanadium, sulphates, PAHs, endotoxins and metals such as iron, copper, nickel, zinc and vanadium, in low- and middle-income countries, poorly designed households using MFBs that have no flues or hood to remove smoke from the living room are often affected by the adverse health effects of PAHs due to lack of ventilation (31).

Health effects

Exposure to wood/biomass smoke (WBSPM) can exacerbate pre-existing respiratory diseases such as asthma and chronic obstructive pulmonary disease (COPD), as well as increase rates of respiratory infections and hospitalisation due to respiratory complications, and an estimated 3 to 4 million deaths per yeare attributable to exposure to the toxic by-products of wood and biomass burning combustion, with countless other minor effects occurring unrecognised (31).

Acute lower respiratory tract infection is a major contributor to the global burden of disease and is also the most common cause of morbidity and mortality, especially in children under five years of age. Almost all of this burden occurs in developing countries, where LRTI is the main source of household energy (32).

Biological recognition and toxicology of biomass exposure

Inhalation of biomass smoke causes inflammation and lung damage, but not much is yet known about how it negatively affects lungs and overall health, common lung toxicity from exposure to biomass and other forms of particulate matter (PM) is due to the ability to: (1) cause oxidative stress through the production of reactive oxygen species, either directly or through enzymatic activation of chemicals in/on PM; (2) deplete antioxidants; (3) modify important macromolecules such as lipids, proteins and DNA through oxidative and non-oxidative processes, and by covalent modification by electrophilic chemicals in/on PM; and (4) activate regulatory molecules such as aryl hydrocarbon (AhR), or scavenger receptors of the innate immune system. However, it is important to note that they have different effects on lung cells and tissues, as well as on human health (33).

Biomass smoke related respiratory diseases

It has been identified that among the more than 200 components present in biomass smoke, some of the most hazardous are carbon monoxide, nitrogen dioxides, sulphur oxides, formaldehyde and polycyclic organic matter. It has therefore been recognised that burning biomass fuels may increase the risk of respiratory disorders such as chronic bronchitis and COPD, asthma, lung cancer, pulmonary fibrosis and tuberculosis (30).

COPD: In most societies, women often play a key role in food preparation in the home, while men are at work or out of the house, globally, it is estimated that almost 50% of COPD deaths in developing countries may be related to biomass exposure, with around 75% of these deaths occurring in women, Available evidence suggests that COPD is the disease most commonly associated with this exposure, and several studies have found that women exposed to cooking smoke are three times more likely to develop COPD in the form of chronic bronchitis than those who cook with cleaner fuels such as electricity or gas (34).

COPD affects one in ten adults worldwide and is among the top three causes of death globally. In 2019, the disease was responsible for the deaths of 3.22 million individuals and there was a 17.5% increase in the number of deaths, with the regions with the highest burden of COPD mortality being Latin America, sub-Saharan Africa, India, China and South-East Asia, according to the Global Burden of Disease study, COPD affected an estimated 104.7 million men and 69.7 million women worldwide over the last decade (35).

Asthma: Asthma is a non-contagious respiratory condition characterised by chronic inflammation of the airways, causing symptoms such as wheezing, chest tightness and coughing. In 2018, approximately 400,000 people died from asthma worldwide. Although numerous studies have been conducted on the relationship between biomass exposure and COPD, little data is available on the association between biomass exposure and asthma. While research results have been conflicting on the relationship between biomass exposure and asthma, evidence is now emerging to suggest that biomass exposure may be related to the risk, prevalence or incidence of asthma (36).

Lung cancer: Lung cancer is the leading cause of cancer-related deaths in developed countries such as North America. This is highlighted by statistics showing that in Canada, for example, more people die from lung cancer than from colorectal, pancreatic and breast cancer combined. By 2020, around 30,000 Canadians are expected to be diagnosed with lung cancer and there are projected to be around 21,000 lung cancer-related deaths. Globally, the cancer burden is projected to double by 2050, with lung cancer at the top of the list (37).

Other respiratory diseases: Exposure to BMF is associated with an interstitial lung disease known as "shack lung". This disease is characterised by carbon accumulation, dust staining and mixed dust fibrosis and has been observed mainly in women chronically exposed to high levels of indoor biomass smoke in developing countries. Bronchial anthracofibrosis has also been reported in older women who have worked long hours in poorly ventilated, smoky kitchens due to incomplete combustion of BMF (38).

3.2 Grounding of the state of the art

3.2.1 Background to nursing interventions in patients with respiratory diseases

During 2018 in a meta-analysis conducted by Sana et al. (39) with the aim of highlighting the relationship between COPD and domestic biomass fuel use in women, with findings that biomass smoke exposure is associated with COPD in women, more attention should be paid to cooking energy and improved cooking cookers in view of the burden faced mainly by women in relation to traditional fuels such as biomass and traditional cooker use, particularly in rural areas.

In a cross-sectional study conducted by Molla et al. (40) in Ethiopia during 2020 in a population of 5830 individuals, the authors determined that respiratory diseases present in this group were related to the use of biomass fuel such as cow dung, presence of burning events, spending time near the cooker during cooking and frequent charcoal cooking, and showed that nursing interventions reduced respiratory conditions due to PAH exposure by improving ventilation, behavioural changes in child handling and cooking patterns.

Nagourney, E et al. (41) in 2020 conducted qualitative research, aiming to characterise disease representations for COPD in a rural community, resulting in interventions that must foster self-efficacy and empowerment by providing tools to enhance self-management and improve connections between people and the health care system, health systems strengthening and continued investment to improve access to treatment are essential, self-management at the household and community level cannot be achieved in a vacuum.

Ken Lee et al. (42) in a systematic review conducted in the UK in 2020 to estimate the regional burden of respiratory diseases caused by biomass exposure, found that people chronically exposed to solid fuels in the home are at increased risk of developing COPD, adding that people chronically exposed to biomass smoke are also at high risk of chronic bronchitis and suggest that nursing interventions and thus urgent integrated health and energy strategies should be strengthened to reduce the adverse health impact of household air pollution.

Fletcher et al (43) in 2020 in a systematic investigation, aiming to identify the factors that experts believe enable the delivery of high quality asthma care, found that well-supported holistic nursing interventions that involve the whole health care system and include the patient voice appear to provide the best outcomes, adding that if substantial improvements in asthma management in primary care are to be achieved globally, combinations of interventions appear to be the most effective.

Valdres et al. (44) during 2020 in an investigation carried out in Spain, with the aim that a nursing plan used in patients with lung cancer can improve the quality of life of the patients gave as a result that nursing plays a crucial role in all phases of the oncological process and, especially, in the final stage of the disease, the work focuses on providing comprehensive and high quality care that ensures the well-being and comfort of the patient and their close environment, whose interventions are focused on preserving the privacy and tranquillity of the patient to guarantee their comfort.

Slang et al. (45) in their literature review conducted during 2020 in Norway aimed to identify and evaluate the evidence base for non-pharmacological or non-technical interventions for breathing difficulties, and to propose interventions that need further research. They found that interventions used to help ICU patients with breathing difficulties showed beneficial effects, some interventions also revealed non-respiratory effects, such as reduction of anxiety and pain, which in turn may contribute to positive respiratory effects.

Sun et al. (46) in 2021 conducted a descriptive research on 157 older adults in China with the aim of determining the effect of breathing-related counselling and nursing on respiratory function, the researchers obtained that for elderly COPD patients, breathing-related counselling and nursing interventions can improve their lung function and respiratory function, alleviate their dyspnoea and sleep disorder, and improve their daily living ability, quality of life and nursing satisfaction.

Sun et al. (47) during 2021 in a descriptive study of 120 patients and with the aim of investigating the impact of the exclusive asthma nursing scheme on the treatment effect of asthma patients determined that with the help of an exclusive asthma nursing scheme asthma patients with asthma can be safely and substantially optimised and their capacity improved, which has a high application value in clinical practice.

In another case-control study conducted by Li Jing et al. (48) during 2022 in China on 96 respiratory medicine patients and aimed to analyse the clinical effectiveness of implementing nursing interventions, the researchers found and concluded that quality nursing interventions to the implementation of conventional care for patients with respiratory diseases can improve patients' clinical symptoms, accelerate their clinical recovery, improve and enhance prognosis and further improve clinical outcomes.

Leonardsen et al. (49) in 2022 conducted a descriptive and exploratory study in Norway with the aim of exploring nurses' perspectives and strategies in patients with respiratory failure, they found that competencies related to observation, assessment and interventions are essential and that nursing strategies included a balance between nursing interventions, medical treatment and a holistic approach to patients' needs.

Zhang et al. (50) conducted a case-control research in 2022, aiming to investigate the efficacy of high-quality nursing care in patients with acute exacerbation of chronic obstructive pulmonary disease, it was found that high-quality nursing intervention has a good therapeutic effect on acute exacerbation of COPD complicated with respiratory failure and added that the establishment of high-quality nursing team, the implementation of safety nursing leads to improve the treatment effect.

In a case study conducted by Hernández et al. (51) during 2022 in Peru, with the aim of improving respiratory conditions in patients through the application of nursing care, it was found that the nursing care process was executed by carrying out a nursing care plan using the NANDA-NOC- NIC trilogy, choosing appropriate interventions in accordance with the problems and/or nursing diagnoses prioritised with the proposed activities based on the identification of human responses.

Rowntree, A et al. (52) in a 2022 study in Australia aimed at determining the effectiveness of care interventions for lung cancer patients, found that interventions improve outcomes among some lung cancer patients and indicate that the effect of these interventions appears to be most relevant in early stage non-small cell lung cancer disease.

Leng, S et al. (53) in a 2022 study conducted in New Mexico to delineate the impact of WS exposure on lung health and mortality in adults aged 40 years or older who ever smoked found that exposure to wood smoke increased the risk of lung cancer incidence and all-cause death, cardiopulmonary diseases and cancers by >50% and shortened lifespan by 3.5 years and concluded that WS exposure as an independent etiological factor for the development of COPD through accelerated decline in lifespan by 3.5 years. 50 % and shortened lifespan by 3.5 years and concluded that exposure to WS as an independent aetiological factor for the development of COPD through accelerated decline of lung function in an obstructive pattern.

In another study by Garg, A et al. (54) on the adverse effects of solid biomass fuel exposure on lung functions, they aimed to assess the effect of solid biomass fuel exposure on lung functions in the non-smoking female population, and found that the cumulative exposure to solid biomass fuel is directly proportional to the severity of lung failure as well as to the severity of symptoms.

Xin et al. (55) in a study conducted during 2022 in China and aimed to explore the perioperative nursing care of lung cancer patients undergoing total pneumonectomy and promote their rehabilitation, determined that nurses should pay more attention to their care and enrich the relevant nursing experience, can improve the perioperative nursing process of total pneumonectomy for lung cancer patients and focus on preoperative airway management.

Pathirathna, M et al. (56) in a study conducted during 2022 in Sri Lanka to examine the relationship between biomass fuel smoke exposure in non-pregnant women of reproductive age in Sri Lanka, found that wood smoke contains several pollutants, including CO, which has the potential to cause systemic inflammation and contributes to respiratory disease.

Shilenje et al. (57) in a 2022 study conducted in Kenya and aimed at documenting the status of biomass fuel use in Kenya, focusing on its effects and consequences, found that BMF use is high, especially in rural areas and informal urban settlements, and cooking with BMF exposes women and young children to harmful indoor air conditions, adding that raising awareness on biomass fuel use among the poor in an effort to minimise biomass use, exposure and associated impacts.

3.3 Conclusions Chapter 1

Nursing interventions are crucial in the management of patients with respiratory diseases associated with exposure to biomass smoke. Nurses play an important role in the prevention, early detection and treatment of these diseases by educating patients and their families about the harmful effects of exposure to biomass smoke, encouraging smoking cessation and promoting healthy lifestyles.

Overall, nursing interventions can improve the quality of life of patients with respiratory diseases associated with biomass smoke exposure by addressing both their physical and psychological needs, promoting self-care and empowering them to take an active role in their care, therefore, nurses should be an integral part of the multidisciplinary team involved in the care of these patients.

Nursing interventions based on Orem's self-care deficit theory can help patients with respiratory diseases associated with biomass smoke exposure to maintain their independence, improve their quality of life and achieve optimal health outcomes, therefore, nurses should consider incorporating this theory into their practice when caring for these patients.

4. CHAPTER II. DIAGNOSIS

4.2 Explanation and presentation of the diagnosis

This research was carried out at the Noboa Parish Health Centre, in the canton of 24 de Mayo in the province of Manabí. The study population used for the development of the present analysis corresponds to those patients with respiratory diseases caused by continuous exposure to biomass smoke, who are regularly seen at this health centre.

Context of the research

According to historians, in the past the parish used to be called "Guineal" due to the presence of vast crops of wild bananas. This led the locals to identify the place as Guineal. However, it is argued that the term derives from the Greek words "Gui", meaning "guineo", and "Neal", meaning "plantation", and when joined together they form "guineo plantation". Subsequently, the Council of Jipijapa took the decision to elevate the status of the village of Guineal to parish through an ordinance. Today, this parish is known as Noboa, in honour of the services rendered by Mr. Diego Noboa in 1822.

The study was carried out at the Noboa Parish Health Centre, which is a locality located in the canton of 24 de Mayo, in the province of Manabí, Ecuador, and lasted from April to June 2023. In order to reach the patients, access was gained to their medical records and then to carry out the survey, informed consent was used for the use of the information provided.

Cases, universe and sample

The Noboa Health Centre has a capacity to attend up to 10,000 inhabitants, the universe is made up of a register of 1,500 people with various illnesses who are attended at the health centre. The final sample participating in this study corresponds to 30 patients between 18 and 75 years of age with respiratory illnesses associated with biomass smoke, who generally come from neighbouring areas, who were chosen and identified through the evaluation of the clinical history provided by the director of the Health Centre.

Design

This study has a quantitative, non-experimental, longitudinal design. An educational guide was developed and educational talks were given after the diagnosis was made, with the aim of educating patients about the dangers of biomass smoke.

Procedure

In order to carry out this research, the cases registered and for which there was a clinical history were investigated, those participants who wanted to participate and were willing to provide information were selected. The sample consisted of 30 people, especially patients located in areas belonging to the parish, materials such as paper and pencil were used for the survey, each contributor was visited in their respective homes where the interview was carried out and the survey was completed, identifying that all the houses used firewood, charcoal and constantly burnt rubbish.

Detailed description

First, we proceeded to talk to the director of the Noboa Parish Health Centre in order to gain access to the records and clinical histories of patients with respiratory diseases. After an exhaustive evaluation, each patient was interviewed in order to ask them if they would be willing to participate in the study, where several affirmative answers were obtained, thus indicating that 30 of the 100 patients would participate in the research.

Subsequently, the first survey was conducted among the patients to determine their knowledge of the respiratory diseases caused by biomass smoke, which was carried out during the month of April 2023, for the collection of data, surveys were used among the participants, which had 11 questions that evaluated their knowledge, This process lasted about a week, as the patients lived in different sectors of the parish. Once the information was collected, the information was processed using a statistical programme called SPSS 25, which was used to obtain answers and determined that the level of understanding of biomass smoke among the inhabitants was nil.

Materials used

A range of traditional and digital materials were used to conduct a survey of nursing interventions in patients with respiratory diseases associated with biomass smoke:

- **Printed questionnaire:** contains the relevant questions on nursing interventions in respiratory diseases associated with biomass smoke, including closed questions to collect qualitative information.

- **Informed consent:** explains the purpose of the survey, how the data is used and the confidentiality of the information collected, participants read and signed this form before participating in the survey.

- **Educational material:** An educational guide on respiratory diseases associated with biomass smoke and recommended nursing interventions was developed.

4.2 Data obtained

In accordance with the results obtained for the elaboration of the research in question, the following results were obtained:

In the first instance, the objectives were answered by means of a survey addressed to the participants; it was found that 100% of the patients surveyed indicated that they did not know what biomass smoke is. The survey described that the nursing staff do not carry out any type of preventive or promotional activity on respiratory diseases associated with biomass smoke aimed at affected patients or the population at risk.

Exposure to smoke was identified by 46.7% of patients as one of the main factors, followed by low socio-economic status (20%), then lack of knowledge about the danger (16.7%) and finally poor access to health services (16.7%).

According to the data obtained from the survey of open questions to the nursing staff, it was determined that 100% have similar criteria, in the first question the total responded that they have a monthly schedule, in question two the staff mentioned that weekly talks are held, in question 3 the 6 graduates interviewed agree that the patients will know more about their illness.

Question 4 also agrees that educational talks help to a great extent to improve patient outcomes. In question 5 which corresponds to the main challenges they answered that the use of scientific language is the most common situation and finally question 6 according to the answers given by the nursing staff they agree that it is necessary due to and that the patients are aware of their work.

4.3 Conclusions of the chapter

Exposure to biomass smoke is the major risk factor for respiratory diseases, people with lifetime exposure to biomass smoke have a high risk of developing COPD, women over 30 years of age who predominantly performed household chores in rural areas have a higher relative risk of COPD, patients' knowledge of this pathology was null in the sample studied.

Nursing activities are necessary as they should assess the patient's exposure history related to biomass smoke, including the type of fuel used for cooking and heating, duration, frequency of exposure, analyse the patient's respiratory symptoms such as coughing, wheezing, shortness of breath, nurses can identify patients at risk and provide appropriate nursing interventions to prevent these diseases.

5. CHAPTER III. PROJECT - PROPOSAL

Educational guide "Respiratory diseases caused by biomass smoke" and talk for users of the Noboa Health Centre".

Respiratory diseases resulting from the inhalation of biomass smoke can have serious consequences for people's quality of life. From acute conditions such as bronchitis and pneumonia, to chronic diseases such as chronic obstructive pulmonary disease (COPD), these diseases can cause uncomfortable symptoms, breathing difficulties and even lead to death.

Given the recognition of the importance of preventing and controlling these diseases, a proposal was drawn up to implement an educational guide and informative talks aimed at all users of the "Noboa" Health Centre. The main objective of this initiative is to provide detailed information on respiratory diseases related to biomass smoke, including their prevention, symptoms and available treatments.

The educational guide is designed to provide comprehensive and accessible material, addressing everything from the harmful effects of biomass smoke to offering practical advice on how to reduce exposure and improve air quality in homes. In addition, the talks will offer the opportunity to interact directly with health professionals, who are available to answer questions and provide personalised guidance.

Context

The proposal focuses specifically on respiratory diseases caused by exposure to biomass smoke from burning wood, charcoal and other solid fuels in enclosed spaces. We will focus on the population of users of the "Noboa" Health Centre as the target group for the educational guide and the informative talks.

The educational guide and information talks are designed to address key aspects of these diseases, including their prevention, symptoms and available treatments. In addition, information is provided on how to reduce exposure to biomass smoke and improve air quality in homes.

By focusing on the users of the "Noboa" Health Centre, the aim is to provide relevant information, tailored to the needs of the local community, with the objective of improving awareness and promoting healthy practices in relation to respiratory diseases caused by biomass smoke.

Sectoral analysis

Respiratory diseases caused by biomass smoke among users of the "Noboa" Health Centre can have negative consequences in terms of awareness, seeking timely medical care, prevention of complications and quality of life, it is essential to address this knowledge gap through educational initiatives to promote respiratory health and improve the wellbeing of users.

The use of biomass smoke in the Noboa parish is very common, as most of the families living in the parish and in neighbouring sectors that receive care at the Health Centre tend to use it for daily activities such as cooking, burning organic material on land for planting and making organic fertilisers, using charcoal to roast meat and other foods, but they do not take into account that the habitual use of this leaves harmful consequences for health and the development of serious respiratory diseases.

Respiratory diseases caused by biomass smoke often have negative impacts on rural dwellers due to the limited availability of clean fuels, unfavourable housing conditions, lack of awareness and education, scarcity of health care services and the impact on quality of life and productivity. It is essential to implement prevention, awareness and access to adequate health care measures to address these negative aspects and protect the respiratory health of rural dwellers.

Given the nature and circumstances of the project, strategies are proposed to achieve the objectives and respond to the suggested proposal, and the following practices are proposed:

- Conduct a knowledge assessment of users, through the use of surveys.
- Implement education strategies such as lectures to educate patients.
- Surveys addressed to nursing staff to verify the nursing strategies applied to users with respiratory diseases.

SWOT analysis

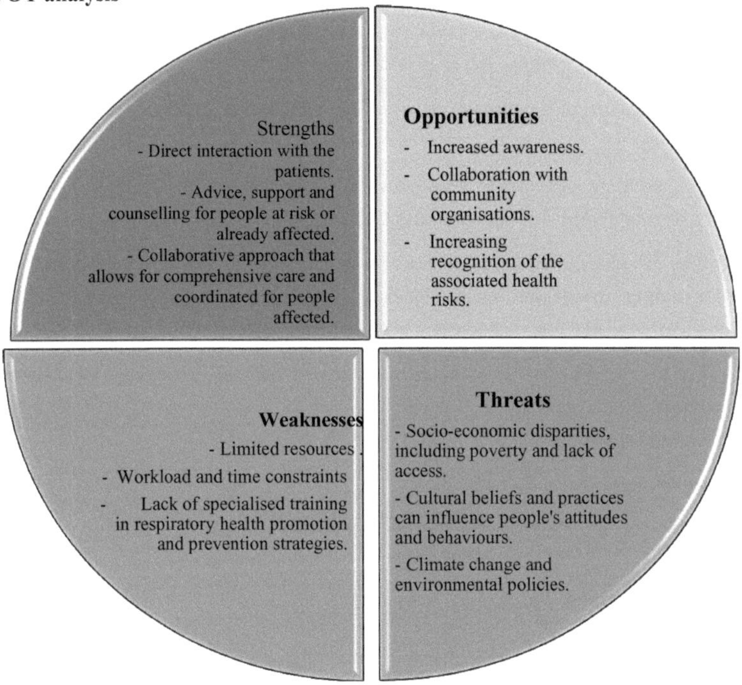

Strengths
- Direct interaction with the patients.
- Advice, support and counselling for people at risk or already affected.
- Collaborative approach that allows for comprehensive care and coordinated for people affected.

Opportunities
- Increased awareness.
- Collaboration with community organisations.
- Increasing recognition of the associated health risks.

Weaknesses
- Limited resources.
- Workload and time constraints
- Lack of specialised training in respiratory health promotion and prevention strategies.

Threats
- Socio-economic disparities, including poverty and lack of access.
- Cultural beliefs and practices can influence people's attitudes and behaviours.
- Climate change and environmental policies.

Methods of implementation

Material and non-material means: Materials:

- Computers
- Data analysis software
- Bibliographic manager
- Visualisation tools for data analysis and presentation

Non-material means

- Funds and financial resources
- Access to scientific literature
- Collaborations with other researchers

Procedure

The organisational procedures carried out to implement the proposal included the following actions:

1. The objectives were identified, established and specified in order to provide preventive education and promote early detection of symptoms in patients.

2. They then assessed 30 medical records and identified needs in the target population to

determine cases of respiratory diseases related to biomass smoke.

3. Once the research sample was established, a survey of patients was conducted to assess their knowledge of biomass smoke and respiratory diseases.

4. Therefore, a survey of the nursing staff and the interventions applied within the Health Centre was analysed.

5. Once the problem concerning respiratory diseases caused by biomass smoke was identified, it was established that the knowledge of the users was null.

6. Therefore, an educational guide on respiratory diseases caused by biomass smoke was developed, including images and logos related to the subject, in order to make the didactic material more dynamic and understandable for the patients of the Health Centre.

7. Finally, a patient survey was conducted to reassess patients' knowledge of respiratory diseases caused by biomass smoke.

Timetable for implementation

Activities/Months	2023					
	January	February	March	April	May	June
Definition of objectives						
Assessment of medical records and determination of study population						
Determination of the sample						
Patient knowledge survey						
Survey of nursing staff						
Definition of knowledge						
Elaboration of an educational guide						
Implementation of educational talks						
Second diagnostic survey of users						

Economic and financial sustainability

This research is economically sustainable, where expenses are covered by the researcher.

Detail	Quantity	P. unitary	P. total
Spheres	5	0,25	1,25
Ream of paper	5	4	20
Draft	6	0,25	1,50
Notebooks	4	0,5	2
Prints	500	0,03	15
Flash memory	1	5	5
Laptop	1	700	700
Mobilisations			300
Texts	1	45	45
Ringed	30	1	30
Refreshments for training	150	1	150
Various			500
Total			$ 1.769

5.1 Conclusions of the chapter

- The development of the educational guide and the delivery of lectures aims to present the risks, harmful effects of exposure to biomass smoke on respiratory health. This allows individuals to recognise the symptoms and take preventive measures to avoid complications.

- The proposal is a valuable strategy to educate, raise awareness, promote respiratory health in the community, by providing accurate and practical information, this initiative has the potential to make a significant difference in people's lives, reducing risks and improving quality of life in relation to respiratory diseases caused by biomass smoke.

6. CHAPTER IV. VALIDATION OF THE PROJECT/PROPOSAL

The validation and implementation of the project involves a thorough review of the educational guide by experts in respiratory health, who ensure the accuracy and timeliness of the information presented. All experts agreed that the educational guide corresponds to the scientific problem.

The experts refer that the educational guide is a proposal with excellent validity to be applied to the institution, staff and patients that conform it and with that avoid the factors that trigger the danger of biomass smoke.

Table (1). Data from the experts

N°	Name and Surname of the Expert	Title Academic	Occupation labour	Validity
1	Dr. Dora Menéndez Macías	Specialist in Pneumology	Pneumologist at Rodriguez Hospital Zambrano	Excellent
2	Dr. Yaritza Quimis Cantos	Specialist in Forensic Medicine, Labour and Nutrition	Medical Specialist, Lecturer at UNESUM.	Excellent
3	Dr. Jorge Jonny Zumba Alban	MSc in Scientific and Epidemiological Research	General Medicine	Excellent
4	Lcda. Estrella Marisol Mero Mg.	Magister in Health management	Nursing teacher at UNESUM.	Excellent
5	Angélica Alcázar Marcillo Mg.	Master's Degree in Nursing in Critical Care	Graduate in Nursing	Excellent

Table (2). Proposal validation instrument.

CONTENT VALIDATION BY EXPERT JUDGEMENT

EDUCATIONAL GUIDE RESPIRATORY DISEASES ASSOCIATED WITH BIOMASS SMOKE

Expert report

Respected Dr, Dr, Lcda, Lcdo: You have been selected to evaluate the educational guide on respiratory diseases associated with biomass smoke which is part of the research entitled: "Nursing interventions in patients with respiratory diseases associated with biomass smoke".

Expert:

Academic degree:

Areas of professional experience: Researcher:

Indicators	**Please indicate your degree of agreement with the following items:** (**1** = strongly disagree; 2 = somewhat disagree; **3** = somewhat agree; **4** = strongly agree)	1	2	3	4
Sufficiency	The content of the educational guide is sufficient to encourage the prevention and promotion of biomass smoke inhalation.				
Functionality	The guide responds to all factors associated with respiratory diseases				
Objectivity	Guidance is expressed in observable behaviours.				
Organisation	The order and content of the educational guide is adequate.				
Clarity	The vocabulary used in the guide is appropriate for the target population to be applied.				
Consistency	The educational guide has a theoretical and scientific basis to support it.				
Coherence	There is coherence between the educational guide and the research problem.				
Importance	The educational guide contributes appropriate information to patients with respiratory diseases.				
Applicability	It considers that the educational guide is applicable for patients and nursing staff.				

EVALUATION CRITERIA OF THE EDUCATIONAL GUIDE

According to the following indicators, evaluate each of the proposed items as appropriate.

Overall evaluation of the educational guide

Content validity of the guide	Excellent	Good	Regular	Deficient

REMARKS:

Reviewed and validated Date:

Signature of the expert

6.1 Analysis of the results

Knowledge survey conducted after the lecture. Table 1. Do you know what biomass smoke is?

Frequency		Percentage	Percentage valid	Cumulative percentage
Valid	Yes	30100,0	100,0	100,0

Source: Researcher

Analysis and interpretation

According to the results of table 1, which refers to the users' knowledge of biomass smoke, 100% of the patients surveyed indicated that they know what biomass smoke is.

Table 2. Has the nursing health staff carried out activities for the promotion and prevention of respiratory diseases caused by biomass smoke?

		Frequency	Percentage	Percentage valid	Cumulative percentage
Valid	Yes	30	100,0	100,0	100,0

Source: Researcher

Analysis and interpretation

As shown in table 2 on whether the nursing staff has educated them about biomass smoke, 100% of the users stated that they have been educated by the staff.

Table 3. What is the relationship between your age and respiratory disease involvement?

		Frequency	Percentage	Percentage valid	Cumulative percentage
Valid	18 30	3	10,0	10,0	10,0
	30 - 50	9	30,0	30,0	40,0
	51 - 75	18	60,0	60,0	100,0
	Total	30	100,0	100,0	

Source: Researcher

Analysis and interpretation

Through table 3 concerning the age of the patients with respiratory disorders, it was determined that 10% of the patients were aged between 18 and 30 years, while 30% were aged between 31 and 50 years and finally 60% of the users indicated that they were older with an age ranging from 51 to 75 years, indicating that the most affected patients are those of older age.

Table 4. Are you exposed to biomass smoke?

Frequency			Percentage	Percentage valid	Cumulative percentage
Valid	Yes	29	96,7	96,7	96,7
	It is not	1	3,3	3,3	100,0
	Total	30	100,0	100,0	

Source: Researcher

Analysis and interpretation

Table 4, which corresponds to and questions patients' exposure to biomass smoke, showed that 96.7% indicated that they were exposed to it, and finally 3.3% indicated that they did not know if they were exposed to biomass smoke.

Table 5. Do you feel irritation or any kind of discomfort when inhaling wood/coal smoke?

Frequency			Percentage	Percentage valid	Cumulative percentage
Valid	Yes	12	40,0	40,0	40,0
	It is not	18	60,0	60,0	100,0
	Total	30	100,0	100,0	

Source: Researcher

Analysis and interpretation

In table 5 corresponding to the presence of any discomfort associated with biomass smoke, 40% of the patients mentioned that they felt discomfort or irritation at respiratory level after some interaction with biomass smoke, finally 60% stated that they did not know if they suffered from any of these symptoms and whether or not they were associated with biomass smoke.

Table 6. What do you do to improve your health?

		Frequency	Percentage	Percentage valid	Cumulative percentage
Valid	**Healthy eating**	6	20,0	20,0	20,0
	None	24	80,0	80,0	100,0
	Total	30	100,0	100,0	

Source: Researcher

Analysis and interpretation

Then, in table 6 which questions the actions that users take to improve their current health status, 80% of the respondents mentioned that they did not do any activity in order to improve their current health status, however, the remaining 20% of the patients showed that they do activities such as eating healthy food in order to lead a healthier lifestyle.

Table 7. Have you ever experienced difficulty or discomfort in breathing?

Frequency			Percentage	Percentage valid	Cumulative percentage
Valid	**Yes**	14	46,7	46,7	46,7
	Sometimes	16	53,3	53,3	100,0
	Total	30	100,0	100,0	

Source: Researcher

Analysis and interpretation

In table 7, which corresponds to the presence of some difficulty or discomfort in breathing, 53.3% of the people indicated that they sometimes had some respiratory discomfort, the remaining 46.7% revealed that they did have breathing difficulties, which demonstrates the existence of cases with respiratory aetiologies.

Table 8. How often do you go to the doctor for respiratory diseases or conditions?

		Frequency	Percentage	Percentage valid	Cumulative percentage
Valid	**Trismistral**	11	36,7	36,7	36,7
	Half-yearly	12	40,0	40,0	76,7
	Annual	7	23,3	23,3	100,0
	Total	30	100,0	100,0	

Source: Researcher

Analysis and interpretation

Through table 8, it was possible to answer the question of interest, which emphasises the frequency with which patients visit the doctor due to the presence of respiratory diseases. 40% indicated that they do so every six months, 36.7% indicated that they do so every three months, and the following 23.3% indicated that they attend annually.

Table 9. Would you like to know about respiratory diseases caused by biomass smoke?

Frequency		Percentage	Percentage valid	Cumulative percentage
Valid	**Yes**	30100,0	100,0	100,0

Source: Researcher

Analysis and interpretation

Table 9, which pertains to the question of whether they would like to obtain information about respiratory diseases associated with biomass smoke, 100% of the participants indicated that they would like to know and acquire more knowledge about this.

Table 10. During the last year, what types of respiratory diseases have you had?

Frequency			Percentage	Percentage valid	Cumulative percentage
Valid	Asthma	4	13,3	13,3	13,3
	Allergy	9	30,0	30,0	43,3
	Influenza	17	56,7	56,7	100,0
	Total	30	100,0	100,0	

Source: Researcher

Analysis and interpretation

Table 10 deals with the type of respiratory diseases diagnosed in the patients, 56.7% indicated that they suffered from influenza, 30% stated that they had suffered from allergies and 13.3% suffered from asthma, which frequently affects this population, coinciding with the data from the first survey.

Which of the following causes do you think influence the development of respiratory diseases associated with biomass smoke?

		Frequency	Percentage	Percentage valid	Cumulative percentage
Valid	Exposure to smoke from wood, coal or manure	14	46,7	46,7	46,7
	Lack of knowledge about the dangers of smoke	5	16,7	16,7	63,3
	Low socio-economic status	6	20,0	20,0	83,3
	Poor access to health services	5	16,7	16,7	100,0
	Total	30	100,0	100,0	

Source: Researcher

Analysis and interpretation

In table 11 on the causes influencing the development of respiratory diseases, 46.7% of patients said that exposure to smoke is one of the main factors, followed by low socio-economic status with 20%, then lack of knowledge about the dangers with 16.7% and finally poor access to health services with 16.7%, similar to the first survey.

6.2 Discussion of the results

Exposure to biomass smoke is a significant problem in rural areas such as Noboa Parish, as the use of fuels such as wood, crop residues, charcoal for cooking and crops is very common, and this prolonged exposure to biomass smoke has serious implications for the respiratory health of people living in these areas.

According to this research and in accordance with the data obtained, nursing interventions play a fundamental role in the prevention and proper use of biomass smoke, the implementation of educational talks and the proposal of a didactic educational guide prepared by the nursing staff is of vital importance as these can be used to implement strategies for prevention, management and recognition of symptoms, as well as helping patients to learn about those practices that are usually carried out and which leave harmful sequelae in people.

The evidence obtained from this research makes it clear that nursing strategies and interventions in patients with respiratory diseases are of great medical relevance, since the interventions carried out during the duration of the project resulted in patients learning more and taking precautionary measures when exposed to smoke, with the aim of reducing this type of diseases or affectations that they suffer in adulthood.

The scientific evidence suggests that patients' knowledge of respiratory diseases is limited, coinciding with the findings obtained, Jam

(58) makes it clear that nurses have multiple roles and responsibility for keeping patients safe in the complex healthcare environment, as well as being responsible for providing knowledge-enhancing interventions. Another study by Mahesh (59) related to knowledge suggests that those living in rural areas are more exposed to increased respiratory diseases associated with biomass smoke especially in the female population, as they are unaware of the adverse effects of smoke use and continue with constant burning and cooking with an oven.

These findings are consistent with research by Becqué (60) which suggests that nursing interventions aimed at supporting family caregivers in end-of-life care at home demonstrate their ability to generate positive outcomes, nurses should combine several components when supporting family caregivers, with the aim of improving their well-being and ability to provide adequate care. This is consistent with Vaismoradi.

(61) which indicates that general guidelines suggest that increasing nurses' knowledge of patient safety, encouraging task collaboration and information sharing, providing regular feedback in the work environment can contribute to improving nurses' adherence to patient safety principles.

The implementation of an educational guide and according to Younas (62) can facilitate or hinder clinical practice by nurses and consequently jeopardise patient safety.

6.3 Conclusions of the chapter

The educational guide, developed in collaboration with respiratory health experts, provides detailed information on the symptoms, causes and treatment options for respiratory diseases related to biomass smoke, also highlights the importance of prevention and offers practical guidelines for reducing exposure to biomass smoke.

The successful implementation and validation of this project depended on collaboration between health professionals, users of the Health Centre and the wider community. Working together with them ensured that the information was delivered effectively and contributed to improving respiratory health awareness and care.

7. GENERAL CONCLUSIONS

It was evident that there was a deficient level of knowledge among users about respiratory diseases associated with biomass smoke, this may be due to a lack of education and awareness of the health risks associated with exposure to this type of smoke, it is important to implement education and dissemination strategies to improve the knowledge of users about these diseases and their implications, since once the project was implemented, the knowledge developed by patients became evident to a large extent.

Nursing activities focused on the promotion and prevention of respiratory diseases associated with biomass smoke were essential for education, and multidisciplinary collaboration is essential to address this health problem effectively and improve the quality of life of those affected.

The main health determinants that influence respiratory diseases associated with biomass smoke are biomass smoke exposure, socio-economic factors, environmental factors, and addressing these determinants in a comprehensive and collaborative manner is essential to prevent and control respiratory diseases in communities exposed to biomass smoke.

Effective education guidance influenced behavioural change towards healthier and safer practices in relation to biomass smoke exposure, by understanding the negative health effects and prevention measures, people can choose to use more efficient cookers, improve the ventilation of their homes and reduce exposure to smoke, which can reduce the risk of respiratory diseases.

8. RECOMMENDATIONS

Providing education and awareness about respiratory diseases associated with biomass smoke is essential, nurses can organise talks, workshops and information sessions in rural communities to inform people about the risks and preventive measures.

Nurses can conduct regular health assessments in rural communities to identify people at risk or showing symptoms of respiratory diseases related to biomass smoke.

Collect relevant demographic data from rural areas where biomass is used as an energy source, including information on socio-economic status, education, access to health services and housing conditions.

Conduct periodic evaluations to determine the effectiveness of the education guide, to gather feedback from users and to measure changes in knowledge and practices.

BIBLIOGRAPHY

1. Myall KJ, Mukherjee B, Castanheira AM, Lam JL, Benedetti G, Mak SM, et al. Persistent post-COVID-19 interstitial lung disease: An observational study of corticosteroid treatment. Ann Am Thorac Soc.2021 May 1 [cited 2023 Apr 26];18(5):799-806. Available from: www.atsjournals.org.

2. Soto D. Intramural pollution from biomass smoke. University and Society. 2022 Feb 22;14(1):396-402.

3. Fandiño-Del-Rio M, Kephart JL, Williams KN, Moulton LH, Steenland NK, Checkley W, et al. Household air pollution exposure and associations with household characteristics among biomass cookstove users in Puno, Peru. Environ Res. 2020 Dec 1;191:110028.

4. WHO. Household air pollution and health [Internet]. 2022 [cited 2023 Apr 26]. Available from: https://www.who.int/es/news-room/fact- sheets/detail/household-air-pollution-and-health

5. WHO. Household air pollution [Internet]. 2022 [cited 2023 Apr 26]. Available from: https://www.who.int/news-room/fact-sheets/detail/household-air-pollution- and-health

6. Ministry of Public Health. Respiratory Diseases: Pneumonia CIE-10J09- J22. Quito-Ecuador; 2021.

7. Callejas De Valero D, Pilay Chávez D, Moreira Vice R, Urdaneta Bracho J, Robles DR, Direction *. Acute respiratory infections in children under 5 years of age at Hospital General Dr. Verdi Cevallos Balda. QhaliKay Journal of Health Sciences ISSN 2588-0608 [Internet]. 2022 Jun 28 [cited 2023 Apr 26];6(2):50-6. Available from: https://revistas.utm.edu.ec/index.php/QhaliKay/article/view/4601/5239

8. Li S, Xu J, Jiang Z, Luo Y, Yang Y, Yu J. Correlation between indoor air pollution and adult respiratory health in Zunyi City in Southwest China: Situation in two different seasons. BMC Public Health [Internet]. 2019 Jun 10 [cited 2023 May 2];19(1):1-14. Available from: https://bmcpublichealth.biomedcentral.com/articles/10.1186/s12889-019-7063-z

9. Shupler M, Hystad P, Birch A, Miller-Lionberg D, Jeronimo M, Arku RE, et al. Household and personal air pollution exposure measurements from 120 communities in eight countries: results from the PURE-AIR study. Lancet Planet Health [Internet]. 2020 Oct 1 [cited 2023 Apr 26];4(10):e451-62. Available from: http://www.thelancet.com/article/S2542519620301972/fulltext

10. Saini J, Dutta M, Marques G. A comprehensive review on indoor air quality monitoring systems for enhanced public health. Sustainable Environment Research [Internet]. 2020 Jan 29 [cited 2023 Apr 26];30(1):1-12. Available from: https://sustainenvironres.biomedcentral.com/articles/10.1186/s42834-020-0047-y

11. Pachauri S, Rao ND, Cameron C. Outlook for modern cooking energy access in Central

America. PLoS One [Internet]. 2018 Jun 1 [cited 2023 Apr 26];13(6):e0197974. Available from: https://journals.plos.org/plosone/article?id=10.1371/journal.pone.0197974

Arturo A, Vasquez A, Antonio D, Marin A, Mateo A, Asesor TC, et al. Prevalence of spirometric alterations related to biomass use in people over 40 years old in the San Pedro del Cebollar neighborhood 2018, Cuenca - Ecuador. 2019 [cited 2023 Apr26]; Available from: http://dspace.uazuay.edu.ec/handle/datos/9432

12. Schilmann A. Air pollution from domestic use of solid fuels and its relation to Chronic Obstructive Pulmonary Disease in the Latin American and Caribbean region. In Mexico: Dirección de Salud Ambiental, Instituto Nacional de Salud Pública; [cited 2023 Apr 26]. Available from:

https://www.paho.org/hq/dmdocuments/2018/2-Dr.-Schilmann-Indoor-Polution- COPD.pdf

13. Fukada M. Nursing Competency: Definition, Structure and Development. Yonago Acta Med. 2018 Mar 28;61(1):001-7.

14. Lupu DE, Aldous A, Anderson E, Schell JO, Groninger H, Sherman MJ, et al. Advance Care Planning Coaching in CKD Clinics: A Pragmatic Randomized Clinical Trial. Am J Kidney Dis [Internet]. 2022 May 1 [cited 2023 Apr 27];79(5):699-708.e1. Available from: https://pubmed.ncbi.nlm.nih.gov/34648897/

15. Meleis A. Theoretical Nursing Development and Progress. 6th Edition, Wolters Kluwer, Philadelphia. - References - Scientific Research Publishing [Internet]. 2018 [cited 2023 Jun 14]. Available from: https://www.scirp.org/%28S%28351jmbntvnsjt1aadkposzje%29%29/reference/ReferencesPapers.aspx?ReferenceID=2776113

16. Walker LO. Gifts of wise women: A reflection on enduring ideas in nursing that transcend time. Nurs Outlook [Internet]. 2020 May 1 [cited 2023 Apr 27];68(3):355-64. Available from: http://www.nursingoutlook.org/article/S0029655419305214/fulltext

17. Riegel B, Jaarsma T, Strömberg A. A middle-range theory of self-care of chronic illness. Advances in Nursing Science [Internet]. 2018 Jul [cited 2023 Apr 27];35(3):194-204. Available from: https://journals.lww.com/advancesinnursingscience/Fulltext/2018/07000/A_Middle_Range_Theory_of_Self_Care_of_Chronic.3.aspx

18. Walker LO. Gifts of wise women: A reflection on enduring ideas in nursing that transcend time. Nurs Outlook [Internet]. 2020 May 1 [cited 2023 Apr 27];68(3):355-64. Available from: http://www.nursingoutlook.org/article/S0029655419305214/fulltext

19. Khademian Z, Kazemi Ara F, Gholamzadeh S. The Effect of Self Care Education Based on Orem's Nursing Theory on Quality of Life and Self-Efficacy in Patients with Hypertension: A Quasi-Experimental Study. Int J Community Based Nurs Midwifery [Internet]. 2020 Apr 1 [cited 2023 Apr 27];8(2):140. Available from:

/pmc/articles/PMC7153422/

20. Hartweg DL, Metcalfe SA. Orem's Self-Care Deficit Nursing Theory: Relevance and Need for Refinement. https://doi.org/101177/08943184211051369 [Internet]. 2021 Dec 23 [cited 2023 Apr 27];35(1):70-6. Available from: https://journals.sagepub.com/doi/10.1177/08943184211051369

21. Brinkman JE, Sharma S. Physiology, Pulmonary. StatPearls [Internet]. 2022 Jul 18 [cited 2023 Apr 26];Available from: https://www.ncbi.nlm.nih.gov/books/NBK482426/

22. National Center for Biotechnology Information (US). Respiratory Diseases - Genes and Disease - NCBI Bookshelf [Internet]. 2023 [cited 2023 Apr 26]. Available from: https://www.ncbi.nlm.nih.gov/books/NBK22167/

23. James SL, Abate D, Abate KH, Abay SM, Abbafati C, Abbasi N, et al. Global, regional, and national incidence, prevalence, and years lived with disability for 354 diseases and injuries for 195 countries and territories, 2018: a systematic analysis for the Global Burden of Disease Study 2018. Lancet [Internet]. 2018 Nov 10 [cited 2023 Apr 26];392(10159):1789-858. Available from: https://pubmed.ncbi.nlm.nih.gov/30496104/

24. Boehm A, Pizzini A, Sonnweber T, Loeffler-Ragg J, Lamina C, Weiss G, et al. Assessing global COPD awareness with Google Trends. Eur Respir J [Internet]. 2019 Jun 1 [cited 2023 Apr 26];53(6). Available from: https://pubmed.ncbi.nlm.nih.gov/31097517/

25. Health indicators. Conceptual and operational aspects. Health indicators. Conceptual and operational aspects. 2018;

26. Balmes JR. When the fetus is exposed to smoke, the developing lung is burned. Am J Respir Crit Care Med [Internet]. 2019 Mar 15 [cited 2023 Apr 26];199(6):684-5. Available from: /pmc/articles/PMC6423106/

27. Garvey C, Criner GJ. Impact of Comorbidities on the Treatment of Chronic Obstructive Pulmonary Disease. Am J Med. 2018 Sep 1;131(9):23-9.

28. Montes de Oca M, Zabert G, Moreno D, Laucho-Contreras ME, Lopez Varela MV, Surmont F. Smoke, Biomass Exposure, and COPD Risk in the Primary Care Setting: The PUMA Study. Respir Care [Internet]. 2018 Aug 1 [cited 2023 Apr 26];62(8):1058-66. Available from: https://rc.rcjournal.com/content/62/8/1058

29. Capistrano SJ, van Reyk D, Chen H, Oliver BG. Evidence of Biomass Smoke Exposure as a Causative Factor for the Development of COPD. Toxics [Internet]. 2018 Dec 1 [cited 2023 Apr 26];5(4). Available from: /pmc/articles/PMC5750564/

30. Taylan O, Kaya D, Bakhsh AA, Demirbas A. Bioenergy life cycle assessment and management in energy generation. Energy Exploration and Exploitation [Internet]. 2018 Jan 1 [cited 2023 Apr 26];36(1):166-81. Available from: https://journals.sagepub.com/doi/full/10.1177/0144598717725871

31. Kayamba V, Zyambo K, Mulenga C, Mwakamui S, Tembo MJ, Shibemba A, et al. Biomass Smoke Exposure Is Associated With Gastric Cancer and Probably Mediated Via

Oxidative Stress and DNA Damage: A Case-Control Study. JCO Glob Oncol [Internet]. 2020 [cited 2023 Apr 27];6:532-41. Available from:

/pmc/articles/PMC7113078/

32. Scott AF, Reilly CA. Wood and Biomass Smoke: Addressing Human Health Risks and Exposures. Chem Res Toxicol [Internet]. 2019 Feb 18 [cited 2023 Apr 27];32(2):219-21. Available from: https://pubs.acs.org/doi/full/10.1021/acs.chemrestox.8b00318

33. Jetmalani K, Thamrin C, Farah CS, Bertolin A, Chapman DG, Berend N, et al. Peripheral airway dysfunction and relationship with symptoms in smokers with

preserved spirometry. Respirology [Internet]. 2018 May 1 [cited 2023 Apr 27];23(5):512-8. Available from: https://onlinelibrary.wiley.com/doi/full/10.1111/resp.13215

34. Halpin DMG, Vogelmeier CF, Agusti A. Lung Health for All: Chronic Obstructive Lung Disease and World Lung Day 2022. Am J Respir Crit Care Med [Internet]. 2022 Sep 15 [cited 2023 Apr 26];206(6):669-71. Available from: https://www.

35. Thakur M, Nuyts PAW, Boudewijns EA, Kim JF, Faber T, Babu GR, et al. Impact of improved cookstoves on women's and child health in low and middle income countries: a systematic review and meta-analysis. Thorax [Internet]. 2018 Nov 1 [cited 2023 Apr 27];73(11):1026-40. Available from: https://thorax.bmj.com/content/73/11/1026

36. Release notice - Canadian Cancer Statistics: A 2020 special report on lung cancer. Health Promot Chronic Dis Prev Can [Internet]. 2020 Sep 1 [cited 2023 Apr 27];40(10):325. Available from: /pmc/articles/PMC7608932/

37. Shah A, Kunal S, Gothi R. Bronchial anthracofibrosis: The spectrum of radiological appearances. Indian J Radiol Imaging [Internet]. 2018 Jul 1 [cited 2023 Apr 27];28(3):333-41.Available from: https://pubmed.ncbi.nlm.nih.gov/30319212/

38. Sana A, Somda SMA, Meda N, Bouland C. Chronic obstructive pulmonary disease associated with biomass fuel use in women: a systematic review and meta-analysis. BMJ Open Respir Res [Internet]. 2018 Jan 1 [cited 2023 Apr 27];5(1):e000246. Available from: https://bmjopenrespres.bmj.com/content/5/1/e000246

39. Adane MM, Alene GD, Mereta ST, Wanyonyi KL. Prevalence and risk factors of acute lower respiratory infection among children living in biomass fuel using households: A community-based cross-sectional study in Northwest Ethiopia. BMC Public Health [Internet]. 2020 Mar 19 [cited 2023 Apr 27];20(1):1-13. Available from:

https://bmcpublichealth.biomedcentral.com/articles/10.1186/s12889-020-08515- w

40. Nagourney EM, Robertson NM, Rykiel N, Siddharthan T, Alupo P, Encarnacion M, et al. Illness representations of chronic obstructive pulmonary disease (COPD) to inform health education strategies and research design-learning from rural Uganda. Health Educ Res [Internet]. 2020 Aug 1 [cited 2023 Apr 27];35(4):258. Available from: /pmc/articles/PMC7787214/

41. Lee KK, Bing R, Kiang J, Bashir S, Spath N, Stelzle D, et al. Adverse health effects associated with household air pollution: a systematic review, meta-analysis, and burden estimation study. Lancet Glob Health [Internet]. 2020 Nov 1 [cited 2023 Apr 27];8(11):e1427-34. Available from: https://pubmed.ncbi.nlm.nih.gov/33069303/

42. Fletcher MJ, Tsiligianni I, Kocks JWH, Cave A, Chunhua C, Sousa JC de, et al. Improving primary care management of asthma: do we know what really works? NPJ Prim Care Respir Med [Internet]. 2020 Dec 1 [cited 2023 Apr 27];30(1). Available from: /pmc/articles/PMC7300034/

43. Valdrés López A, Marín Zarza M, Bruna Barranco I, Martínez Giménez L. Nursing care plan for patients with end-stage lung cancer. Revista Sanitaria de Investigación, ISSN-e 2660-7085, Vol 1, Nº 8, 2020 [Internet]. 2020 [cited 2023 Apr 27];1(8):4. Available from: https://dialnet.unirioja.es/servlet/articulo?codigo=7653027&info=resumen&idio ma=SPA

44. Slang R, Finsrud LT, Olsen BF. Nursing interventions in intensive care unit patients with breathing difficulties: A scoping review of the evidence. Nord J Nurs Res [Internet]. 2020 Dec 1 [cited 2023 May 8];40(4):176-87. Available from: https://journals.sagepub.com/doi/full/10.1177/2057158520948834

45. Sun X, Shen Y, Shen J. Respiration-related guidance and nursing can improve the respiratory function and living ability of elderly patients with chronic obstructive pulmonary disease. Am J Transl Res [Internet]. 2021 May 30 [cited 2023 Apr 27];13(5):4686. Available from: /pmc/articles/PMC8205811/

46. Sun Y, Sun F, Lin C, Wang F. The impact of asthma-exclusive nursing scheme on the treatment effect of asthma patients. Am J Transl Res [Internet]. 2021 [cited 2023 Apr 27];13(8):9048. Available from: /pmc/articles/PMC8430090/

47. Wu LJ, Jiao WW, Wang HH, Li G, Li P, Wang SJ. Analysis of the Effectiveness of Nursing Interventions in Critically Ill Patients in Respiratory Medicine. J Healthc Eng. 2022;2022.

48. Leonardsen AC, Gulbrandsen T, Wasenius C, Fossen LT. Nursing perspectives and strategies in patients with respiratory insufficiency. Nurs Crit Care [Internet]. 2022 Jan 1 [cited 2023 Apr 27];27(1):27-35. Available from: https://onlinelibrary.wiley.com/doi/full/10.1111/nicc.12555

49. Zhang J, Xu N, Zheng D. Effect of High-Quality Nursing Care on Patients with Acute Exacerbation of Chronic Obstructive Pulmonary Disease Complicated with Respiratory Failure: An Observational Cohort Study. Appl Bionics Biomech [Internet]. 2022 [cited 2023 Apr 27];2022. Available from:

/pmc/articles/PMC9208997/

50. Quijandria MCH, Apaza EH, Guado NC, Condori MY. Nursing care process applied to the mature adult with pneumonia and respiratory failure post COVID-19. Investigación e Innovación: Revista Científica de Enfermería [Internet]. 2022 May 24 [cited 2023 Apr

27];2(1):162-72. Available from: https://revistas.unjbg.edu.pe/index.php/iirce/article/view/1394/1681

51. Rowntree RA, Hosseinzadeh H. Lung Cancer and Self-Management Interventions: A Systematic Review of Randomised Controlled Trials. Int J Environ Res Public Health [Internet]. 2022 Jan 1 [cited 2023 May 8];19(1). Available from: /pmc/articles/PMC8744740/

52. Leng S, Picchi MA, Meek PM, Jiang M, Bayliss SH, Zhai T, et al. Wood smoke exposure affects lung aging, quality of life, and all-cause mortality in New Mexican smokers. Respir Res [Internet]. 2022 Dec 1 [cited 2023 May 8];23(1):1-15. Available from: https://respiratory-research.biomedcentral.com/articles/10.1186/s12931-022-02162-y

53. Garg A, Bagri S, Choudhary P, Singh D, Gupta M, Gaur S. The adverse effects of solid biomass fuel exposure on lung functions in non-smoking female population. J Family Med Prim Care [Internet]. 2022 [cited 2023 May 8];11(6):2499. Available from: https://journals.lww.com/jfmpc/Fulltext/2022/06000/The_adverse_effects_of_solid_biomass_fuel_exposure.39.aspx

54. Xin Z, Tu K, Wu H, Li C, Zhong J, Xin Z, et al. Perioperative Nursing Care for Patients with Lung Cancer Undergoing Total Pneumonectomy. J Cancer Ther [Internet]. 2022 Apr 6 [cited 2023 May 8];13(4):234-41. Available from: http://www.scirp.org/journal/PaperInformation.aspx?PaperID=116866

55. Pathirathna ML, Samarasekara BPP, Mendis C, Dematawewa CMB, Sekijima K, Sadakata M, et al. Is biomass fuel smoke exposure associated with anemia in non-pregnant reproductive-aged women? PLoS One [Internet]. 2022 Aug 1 [cited 2023 May 8];17(8):e0272641. Available from: https://journals.plos.org/plosone/article?id=10.1371/journal.pone.0272641

56. Shilenje ZW, Maloba S, Ongoma V. A review on household air pollution and biomass use over Kenya. Front Environ Sci. 2022 Nov 8;10:2190.

57. Jam R, Mesquida J, Hernández Ó, Sandalinas I, Turégano C, Carrillo E, et al. Nursing workload and compliance with non-pharmacological measures to prevent ventilator-associated pneumonia: a multicentre study. Nurs Crit Care [Internet]. 2018 Nov 1 [cited 2023 Jun 14];23(6):291-8. Available from: https://pubmed.ncbi.nlm.nih.gov/30182383/

58. Mahesh PA, Lokesh KS, Madhivanan P, Chaya SK, Jayaraj BS, Ganguly K, et al. The Mysuru stUdies of Determinants of Health in Rural Adults (MUDHRA), India. Epidemiol Health [Internet]. 2018 [cited 2023 Jun 14];40:e2018027. Available from: http://www.e-epih.org/journal/view.php?doi=10.4178/epih.e2018027.

59. Becqué YN, Rietjens JAC, van Driel AG, van der Heide A, Witkamp E. Nursing

interventions to support family caregivers in end-of-life care at home: A systematic narrative review. Int J Nurs Stud. 2019 Sep 1;97:28-39.

60. Vaismoradi M, Tella S, Logan PA, Khakurel J, Vizcaya-Moreno F. Nurses' Adherence to Patient Safety Principles: A Systematic Review. International Journal of Environmental Research and Public Health 2020, Vol 17, Page 2028 [Internet]. 2020 Mar 19 [cited 2023 Jun 14];17(6):2028. Available from: https://www.mdpi.com/1660-4601/17/6/2028/htm

61. Younas A, Quennell S. Usefulness of nursing theory-guided practice: an integrative review. Scand J Caring Sci [Internet]. 2019 Sep 1 [cited 2023 Jun 14];33(3):540-55. Available from: https://onlinelibrary.wiley.com/doi/full/10.1111/scs.12670

ANNEXES

Annex 1. Survey applied to patients in Noboa Parish.

Data

Province: **Canton:**

Year: **Date:**

Objective:

Instructions: Mark with an X as appropriate.

1. **Do you know what biomass smoke is?**

Yes_

No _

2. **Has the nursing staff carried out activities for the promotion and prevention of respiratory diseases caused by biomass smoke?**

Yes_

No _

3. **What is the relationship between your age and the occurrence of respiratory diseases?**

18 to 30 years old ____________________

30 to 50 years ________________________

51 to 75 years ________________________

4. **Are you exposed to biomass smoke?**

Yes_ No____________________ No se____

5. **Do you feel irritation or discomfort when inhaling wood/coal smoke?**

Yes ______________

No ______________No se_____

6. **What are you doing to improve your health?**

Physical activity ________________________

Healthy eating ______________________________

None______________________________

7. **Have you ever had difficulty or discomfort in breathing?**

Yes_ No ____________________

Sometimes______________________________

8. How often do you see a doctor for respiratory diseases or conditions?

Weekly______________________________

Quarterly______________________________

Semi-annually______________________________

Annually______________________________

Never______________________________

9. Would you like to know about respiratory diseases caused by biomass smoke?

Yes_ **No _____**

10. During the last year, what types of respiratory illnesses have you had?

Asthma______________________________ -----

Allergy______________________________

Influenza______________________________

11. Which of the following causes do you think influence the development of respiratory diseases associated with biomass smoke?

Exposure to smoke from wood, charcoal or manure__

Lack of knowledge about the dangers of smoke______________________

Low socio-economic status ____________________

Poor access to health services ________________________

Annex 2. Interview model applied to the staff of the Noboa Health Centre.

THEME: Nursing interventions in patients with respiratory diseases associated with biomass smoke.

1.- Do you have a daily training schedule for users?

2.- How often do you give educational talks to users?

3.- Do you think it is important to give educational talks to users?

4.- Do you think that educational talks can help improve patient health outcomes?

5.- What challenges have you faced in providing educational talks to patients and how have you overcome them?

6.- Do you think it is necessary or important to educate the patient on the subject of biomass smoke?

Informed consent or assent

I, Lorena María Loor Alvarado, a graduate in Nursing and currently a student of the Master's Degree in Care Management at the Faculty of Health Sciences of the UNESUM Postgraduate Institute, can be contacted on my mobile number: 0989651683 or write an email to lorenaloor99@gmail.com. I am conducting research entitled "Nursing interventions in patients with respiratory diseases associated with biomass smoke", the objective of which is to evaluate the effectiveness of nursing interventions through the promotion and prevention of respiratory diseases associated with biomass smoke.

Your participation is completely voluntary, feel free to decide, however, you were chosen to take part in this study because you meet the criteria of interest for the development of this research. Therefore, for the development of this research, information must be collected by filling in a questionnaire that includes the following topics: a survey will be carried out on the topics related to the research.

Feel free to ask questions if you do not understand; if required, ask for a copy of this document. When you have understood the information and have decided to participate voluntarily, the consent will be handled in person with the respective signatures of the participant.

The data provided will be analysed and the results of the study will be presented at a meeting, pandemic conditions permitting, informing you in a timely manner of the day and time when the results will be shared.

GUARANTEES OF THEIR PARTICIPATION

The information you provide when completing the questionnaires will be kept strictly confidential, no personal information (name, address, ID) will be requested from you, nor will your name be used in the research.

There is no cost to you to participate in this study; nor will you receive any financial compensation for participation. Since your participation is voluntary, you are free to withdraw from this study if you choose to do so, without any reprisal or limitation on the services and care you receive here.

The data obtained will be kept by the researcher for a period of 7 years as stipulated in Art. 10 (a) of the regulations in force in Ecuador, where it mentions that: Facilities that allow work to be carried out under conditions of safety, security and confidentiality are to be maintained.

confidentiality, with appropriate space for the Secretariat of the Committee and for meetings, as well as for the handling and archiving of confidential documents, which shall be stored for a period of seven (7) years. and shall only be used for academic purposes, the results shall be disseminated at scientific events and published in scientific journals only.

The information obtained from the application of the questionnaires will be used only for the purpose of validating the psychoeducational programme and will be handled confidentially. The researcher linked to the proposal, whose details are noted below, will be available to answer questions before, during and after the conclusion of the psychoeducational programme proposal.

Thank you in advance for your valuable collaboration in the development of this study. By signing the consent form you agree to participate voluntarily in this proposed intervention.

I____have read the information provided or read to me and understood the contents of this document, all my doubts have been answered and I know that I can withdraw at any time I wish; therefore I have received sufficient information and voluntarily agree to participate in this research.

I understand the risks and benefits and therefore give my consent to participate in the research study summarized on this form. I understand that, if I do not agree, it will not affect the care I receive at this or any other health care institution.

Participant's Signature

DateDay/month/year

I have explained the study to the above participant and confirmed their understanding for informed consent.

________ __________

Signature of the researcher Date

VALIDACIÓN DE CONTENIDO POR JUICIO DE EXPERTOS

GUÍA EDUCATIVA ENFERMEDADES RESPIRATORIAS ASOCIADAS AL HUMO DE BIOMASA

Informe de experto

Respetable Dra. Usted ha sido seleccionado para evaluar la guia educativa sobre las enfermedades respiratorias asociadas al humo de biomasa que forma parte de la investigación denominada: "Intervenciones de enfermería en pacientes con enfermedades respiratorias asociadas al humo de biomasa"

Experto: Dra. Dora Menéndez Macias

Grado Académico: Especialista en Neumología

Áreas de experiencia: Directora Medica del Hospital Rodríguez Zambrano, Neumóloga del Hospital Rodríguez Zambrano

Investigador: Licenciada en Enfermería. Lorena María Loor Alvarado

Indicadores	Indique su grado de acuerdo frente a los siguientes ítems: (1 = muy en desacuerdo, 2 = algo en desacuerdo; 3 = algo de acuerdo; 4 = muy de acuerdo)	1	2	3	4
Suficiencia	El contenido de la guía educativa es suficiente para fomentar la prevención y promoción de la inhalación del humo de biomasa.				X
Funcionalidad	La guía responde a todos los factores asociados a las enfermedades respiratorias				X
Objetividad	La guía esta expresada en comportamientos observables.				X
Organización	El orden y contenido de la guía educativa es adecuado.				X
Claridad	El vocabulario empleado en la guía es adecuado para la población diana a aplicar.				X
Consistencia	La guía educativa tiene base teórica y científica que la respaldan.				X

Coherencia	Existe coherencia entre la guía educativa y el problema de investigación.	X
Importancia	La guía educativa contribuye información adecuada a los pacientes con enfermedades respiratorias	X
Aplicabilidad	Considera que la guía educativa es aplicable para los pacientes y el personal de enfermería.	X

CRITERIOS DE EVALUACIÓN DE LA GUÍA EDUCATIVA

De acuerdo con los siguientes indicadores evalúe cada uno de los ítems propuestos según corresponda.

Evaluación general de la guía educativa

Validez de contenido de la guía	Excelente	Buena	Regular	Deficiente
	X			

OBSERVACIONES:

Ninguna

Revisado y validado

Fecha: 11 de julio del 2023

Firma del expérto

Ministerio de Salud Publica
Hospital Rodriguez Zambrano
Dra. Dora Menéndez M.
NEUMÓLOGA
C.I. 1309473468
REG. SENESCYT:7174R-15-24596

Dra. Dora Menéndez Macias

C.I 1309473468

VALIDACIÓN DE CONTENIDO POR JUICIO DE EXPERTOS

GUÍA EDUCATIVA ENFERMEDADES RESPIRATORIAS ASOCIADAS AL HUMO DE BIOMASA

Informe de experto

Respetable Dra. Usted ha sido seleccionado para evaluar la guía educativa sobre las enfermedades respiratorias asociadas al humo de biomasa que forma parte de la investigación denominada: "Intervenciones de enfermería en pacientes con enfermedades respiratorias asociadas al humo de biomasa"

Experto: Dra. Yaritza Quimis Cantos

Grado Académico: Especialista en Medicina Legal, Laboral y Nutrición

Áreas de experiencia: Docente en la Universidad Estatal del Sur de Manabí

Investigador: Licenciada en Enfermería. Lorena María Loor Alvarado

Indicadores	Indique su grado de acuerdo frente a los siguientes ítems: (1 = muy en desacuerdo; 2 = algo en desacuerdo; 3 = algo de acuerdo; 4 = muy de acuerdo)	1	2	3	4
Suficiencia	El contenido de la guía educativa es suficiente para fomentar la prevención y promoción de la inhalación del humo de biomasa.				X
Funcionalidad	La guía responde a todos los factores asociados a las enfermedades respiratorias				X
Objetividad	La guía esta expresada en comportamientos observables.				X
Organización	El orden y contenido de la guía educativa es adecuado.				X
Claridad	El vocabulario empleado en la guía es adecuado para la población diana a aplicar.				X
Consistencia	La guía educativa tiene base teórica y científica que la respaldan.				X
Coherencia	Existe coherencia entre la guía educativa y el problema de investigación.				X

Importancia	La guía educativa contribuye información adecuada a los pacientes con enfermedades respiratorias.	X
Aplicabilidad	Considera que la guía educativa es aplicable para los pacientes y el personal de enfermería.	X

CRITERIOS DE EVALUACIÓN DE LA GUÍA EDUCATIVA

De acuerdo con los siguientes indicadores evalúe cada uno de los ítems propuestos según corresponda.

Evaluación general de la guía educativa

Validez de contenido de la guía	**Excelente**	**Buena**	**Regular**	**Deficiente**
	X			

OBSERVACIONES:

Ninguna

Revisado y validado

Fecha: 27 de Junio del 2023

Firma del experto

Dra. Yaritza Quimis Cantos

VALIDACIÓN DE CONTENIDO POR JUICIO DE EXPERTOS

GUÍA EDUCATIVA ENFERMEDADES RESPIRATORIAS ASOCIADAS AL HUMO DE BIOMASA

Informe de experto

Respetable Dr.: Usted ha sido seleccionado para evaluar la guía educativa sobre las enfermedades respiratorias asociadas al humo de biomasa que forma parte de la investigación denominada: "Intervenciones de enfermería en pacientes con enfermedades respiratorias asociadas al humo de biomasa"

Experto: Médico Cirujano. Jorge Jonny Zumba Albán

Grado académico: Magister en Investigación Científica y Epidemiológica

Áreas de experiencia profesional: Hospital Básico Jipijapa, IESS Jipijapa, Docente en la Universidad Estatal del Sur de Manabí

Investigador: Licenciada en Enfermería. Lorena María Loor Alvarado

Indicadores	Indique su grado de acuerdo frente a los siguientes ítems: (1 = muy en desacuerdo; 2 = algo en desacuerdo; 3 = algo de acuerdo; 4 = muy de acuerdo)	1	2	3	4
Suficiencia	El contenido de la guía educativa es suficiente para fomentar la prevención y promoción de la inhalación del humo de biomasa.				X
Funcionalidad	La guía responde a todos los factores asociados a las enfermedades respiratorias				X
Objetividad	La guía esta expresada en comportamientos observables.			X	
Organización	El orden y contenido de la guía educativa es adecuado.				X
Claridad	El vocabulario empleado en la guía es adecuado para la población diana a aplicar.				X
Consistencia	La guía educativa tiene base teórica y científica que la respaldan.				X

Coherencia	Existe coherencia entre la guía educativa y el problema de investigación.	X
Importancia	La guía educativa contribuye información adecuada a los pacientes con enfermedades respiratorias.	X
Aplicabilidad	Considera que la guía educativa es aplicable para los pacientes y el personal de enfermería.	X

CRITERIOS DE EVALUACIÓN DE LA GUÍA EDUCATIVA

De acuerdo con los siguientes indicadores evalúe cada uno de los ítems propuestos según corresponda.

Evaluación general de la guía educativa

Validez de contenido de la guía	Excelente	Buena	Regular	Deficiente
	X			

OBSERVACIONES:

Ninguna

Revisado y validado

Fecha: 17 de junio del 2023

Firma del experto

CI: 1703976657

VALIDACIÓN DE CONTENIDO POR JUICIO DE EXPERTOS

GUÍA EDUCATIVA ENFERMEDADES RESPIRATORIAS ASOCIADAS AL HUMO DE BIOMASA

Informe de experto

Respetable Mg. Lcda.: Usted ha sido seleccionado para evaluar la guía educativa sobre las enfermedades respiratorias asociadas al humo de biomasa que forma parte de la investigación denominada: "Intervenciones de enfermería en pacientes con enfermedades respiratorias asociadas al humo de biomasa"

Experto: Lcda. Estrella Marisol Mero

Grado académico: Magister en Gerencia en Salud

Áreas de experiencia profesional: Docente

Investigador: Lcda. Lorena María Loor Alvarado

Indicadores	Indique su grado de acuerdo frente a los siguientes ítems: (1 = muy en desacuerdo; 2 = algo en desacuerdo; 3 = algo de acuerdo; 4 = muy de acuerdo)	1	2	3	4
Suficiencia	El contenido de la guía educativa es suficiente para fomentar la prevención y promoción de la inhalación del humo de biomasa.				X
Funcionalidad	La guía responde a todos los factores asociados a las enfermedades respiratorias				X
Objetividad	La guía esta expresada en comportamientos observables.				X
Organización	El orden y contenido de la guía educativa es adecuado.			X	
Claridad	El vocabulario empleado en la guía es adecuado para la población diana a aplicar.				X
Consistencia	La guía educativa tiene base teórica y científica que la respaldan.				X
Coherencia	Existe coherencia entre la guía educativa y el problema de investigación.				X

	con enfermedades respiratorias.	
Aplicabilidad	Considera que la guía educativa es aplicable para los pacientes y el personal de enfermería.	X

CRITERIOS DE EVALUACIÓN DE LA GUÍA EDUCATIVA

De acuerdo con los siguientes indicadores evalúe cada uno de los ítems propuestos según corresponda.

Evaluación general de la guía educativa

Validez de contenido de la guía	Excelente	Buena	Regular	Deficiente
	X			

OBSERVACIONES:

Ninguna

Revisado y validado

Fecha: 17 de junio del 2023

Firma del experto

DOCENTE UNESUM

REG. Senescyt: 1031 08-6754

VALIDACIÓN DE CONTENIDO POR JUICIO DE EXPERTOS

GUÍA EDUCATIVA ENFERMEDADES RESPIRATORIAS ASOCIADAS AL HUMO DE BIOMASA

Informe de experto

Respetable Mg. Lcda.: Usted ha sido seleccionado para evaluar la guia educativa sobre las enfermedades respiratorias asociadas al humo de biomasa que forma parte de la investigación denominada: "Intervenciones de enfermería en pacientes con enfermedades respiratorias asociadas al humo de biomasa"

Experto: Mg. Angélica Adriana Alcázar Marcillo

Grado académico: Magister en Mención en Enfermería En Cuidados Intensivos

Investigador: Lcda. Lorena María Loor Alvarado

Indicadores	Indique su grado de acuerdo frente a los siguientes ítems: (1 = muy en desacuerdo; 2 = algo en desacuerdo; 3 = algo de acuerdo; 4 = muy de acuerdo)	1	2	3	4
Suficiencia	El contenido de la guía educativa es suficiente para fomentar la prevención y promoción de la inhalación del humo de biomasa.				X
Funcionalidad	La guia responde a todos los factores asociados a las enfermedades respiratorias				X
Objetividad	La guia esta expresada en comportamientos observables.				X
Organización	El orden y contenido de la guia educativa es adecuado.				X
Claridad	El vocabulario empleado en la guía es adecuado para la población diana a aplicar.				X
Consistencia	La guia educativa tiene base teórica y científica que la respaldan.				X
Coherencia	Existe coherencia entre la guia educativa y el problema de investigación.				X

Importancia	La guía educativa contribuye información adecuada a los pacientes con enfermedades respiratorias.	X
Aplicabilidad	Considera que la guia educativa es aplicable para los pacientes y el personal de enfermeria.	X

CRITERIOS DE EVALUACIÓN DE LA GUÍA EDUCATIVA

De acuerdo con los siguientes indicadores evalúe cada uno de los ítems propuestos según corresponda.

Evaluación general de la guía educativa

Validez de contenido de la guía	Excelente	Buena	Regular	Deficiente
	X			

OBSERVACIONES:

Ninguna

Revisado y validado

Fecha: 27 de junio del 2023

Firma del experto

Lcda. Angélica Alcázar Mg.

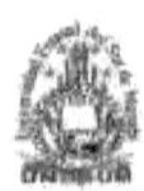

UNIVERSIDAD ESTATAL DEL SUR DE MANABI
Creada el 7 de febrero del 2001, según Registro Oficial # 261
CENTRO DE IDIOMAS

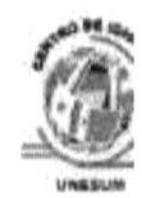

CERTIFICADO No. 591.

Lic.
Mercedes Lucas Chóez
COORDINADORA DE LA MAESTRIA EN GESTION DEL CUIDADO– POSTGRADO - UNESUM
En su despacho.-

De mi consideración:

Por medio de la presente me permito CERTIFICAR que fue corregido el Summary, correspondiente a la Tesis de Grado **"INTERVENCIONES DE ENFERMERÍA EN PACIENTES CON ENFERMEDADES RESPIRATORIAS ASOCIADAS AL HUMO DE BIOMASA,"** Previo a la obtención del título de Magister en Gestión del Cuidado al maestrante, **Lorena María Loor Alvarado,** mismo que fue corregido por la Lic. Gloria Pincay Rodríguez, Mg. Eii.

Particular que hago extensivo para los fines consiguientes.

Jipijapa, 27 de Junio del 2023.

Atentamente,

UNIVERSIDAD ESTATAL DEL SUR DE MANABÍ
UNESUM
CENTRO DE IDIOMAS
JIPIJAPA - MANABÍ

Lic. Paola Yadira Moreira Aguayo, Mg. Eii.
COORDINADORA DEL CENTRO DE IDIOMAS

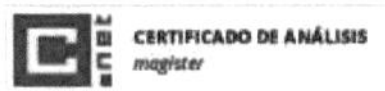

CERTIFICADO DE ANÁLISIS
magister

Proyecto de titulacion - Autora Lcda Lorena Maria Loor Alvarado - Tutora Mg Virginia Pincay Pin (1)

3% Similitudes

< 1% Texto entre comillas
< 1% similitudes entre comillas
2% Idioma no reconocido

Nombre del documento: Proyecto de titulacion - Autora Lcda Lorena Maria Loor Alvarado - Tutora Mg Virginia Pincay Pin (1).pdf
ID del documento: 4530f64c3e0c41b8fb2453aa7b06057c16378f7c
Tamaño del documento original: 2,31 MB

Depositante: Pincay Virginia
Fecha de depósito: 4/7/2023
Tipo de carga: interface
fecha de fin de análisis: 4/7/2023

Número de palabras: 17.790
Número de caracteres: 125.503

Ubicación de las similitudes en el documento:

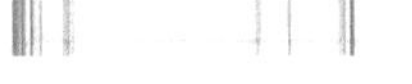

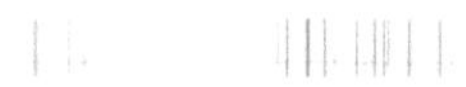

Fuentes principales detectadas

Nº	Descripciones	Similitudes	Ubicaciones	Datos adicionales
1	repositorio.unesum.edu.ec http://repositorio.unesum.edu.ec/bitstream/53000/4206/1/Tesis Katty Tumbaco.pdf 2 fuentes similares	1%		Palabras idénticas : 1% (218 palabras)
2	dspace.utb.edu.ec | Inhalación del humo de biomasa y su incidencia en las enferme... http://dspace.utb.edu.ec:8080/jspui/bitstream/49000/2381/6/P-UTB-FCS-TERR-000007.pdf.txt 1 fuente similar	< 1%		Palabras idénticas : < 1% (157 palabras)
3	dspace.utb.edu.ec http://dspace.utb.edu.ec/bitstream/handle/49000/2381/P-UTB-FCS-TERR-000007.pdf	< 1%		Palabras idénticas : < 1% (113 palabras)
4	www.ncbi.nlm.nih.gov | Household air pollution and COPD: cause and effect or con... https://www.ncbi.nlm.nih.gov/pmc/articles/PMC8888958/ 8 fuentes similares	< 1%		Palabras idénticas : < 1% (72 palabras)
5	[illegible] https://dspace.ucacue.edu.ec/bitstream/ucacue/8596/3/9BT2019-MTI174.pdf.txt 5 fuentes similares	< 1%		Palabras idénticas : < 1% (69 palabras)

Fuentes con similitudes fortuitas

Nº	Descripciones	Similitudes	Ubicaciones	Datos adicionales
1	pubmed.ncbi.nlm.nih.gov | Peripheral airway dysfunction and relationship with sym... https://pubmed.ncbi.nlm.nih.gov/29141272/	< 1%		Palabras idénticas : < 1% (10 palabras)
2	www.ncbi.nlm.nih.gov | Illness representations of chronic obstructive pulmonary di... https://www.ncbi.nlm.nih.gov/pmc/articles/PMC7787214	< 1%		Palabras idénticas : < 1% (10 palabras)

Fuentes ignoradas

Estas fuentes han sido retiradas del cálculo del porcentaje de similitud por el propietario del documento.

Nº	Descripciones	Similitudes	Ubicaciones	Datos adicionales
1	Proyecto de titulacion - Autora Lcda Lorena Maria Loor Alvarado - Tutora ... #d27b63 El documento proviene de mi biblioteca de referencias	84%		Palabras idénticas : 84% (15.786 palabras)
2	Tesis de fabricio rivera - corr.docx | Tesis de fabricio rivera - corr #4081d5 El documento proviene de mi grupo	< 1%		Palabras idénticas : < 1% (152 palabras)
3	Tesis de fabricio rivera - corr.docx | Tesis de fabricio rivera - corr #80d5c7 El documento proviene de mi grupo	< 1%		Palabras idénticas : < 1% (152 palabras)
4	www.mdpi.com | IJERPH | Free Full-Text | Nurses' Adherence to Patient Safety Princi... https://www.mdpi.com/1660-4601/17/6/2028/htm	< 1%		Palabras idénticas : < 1% (30 palabras)

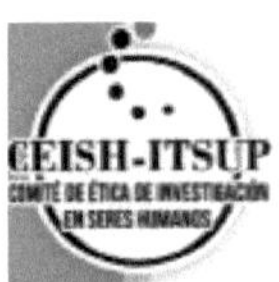

Para:
Lorena María Loor Alvarado-Investigador Principal
CC:
Virginia Esmeralda Pincay Pin

Título del Protocolo: Intervenciones de enfermería en pacientes con enfermedades respiratorias asociadas al humo de biomasa en la Parroquia Noboa Abril - Junio 2023.
Protocolo #: 1675717227
Versión: 1
Fecha de recepción: 06/02/2023
Código CEISH ITSUP: CEISH-ITSUP.010 – 2023

Por medio de la presente se certifica que el estudio de investigación **"Intervenciones de enfermería en pacientes con enfermedades respiratorias asociadas al humo de biomasa en la Parroquia Noboa Abril - Junio 2023."** fue avalado por el Comité de Ética de Investigación en Seres Humanos (CEISH) del ITSUP, el mismo que una vez cumplido satisfactoriamente la fase investigativa se da por finalizada la investigación.

Certifico que la información contenida en este documento es veraz y que esta investigación se ejecutó de conformidad con el proyecto de investigación aprobado por el CEISH ITSUP.

Cualquier pregunta, correspondencia y formas, envíelas al correo electrónico del CEISH ITSUP: comité.etica@itsup.edu.ec

Cordialmente,

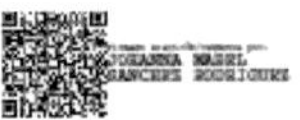

Dra. Mabel Sánchez Rodríguez
Presidente del Comité de Ética de Investigación en Seres Humanos (CEISH)

(03/07/2023)
Fecha de Correspondencia

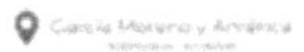
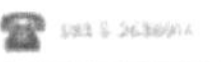
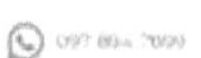
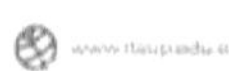
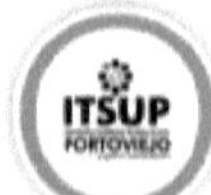

SOUTHERN STATE UNIVERSITY OF MANABÍ

Created on February 7, 2001, *according to Official Registry No. 261 HIGHER ACADEMIC COLLEGATE BODY*

FORM OF:

AUTHORISATION OF PUBLICATION RIGHTS IN THE UNESUM I N S T I T U T U T IO N A L DIGITAL REPOSITORY

The undersigned, Lorena Maria Loor Alvarado, as author of the following written work entitled "**Nursing interventions in patients with respiratory diseases associated with biomass smoke**", grants the Universidad Estatal del Sur de Manabí, free of charge and non-exclusively, the rights of reproduction and public distribution of the work, which constitutes a work of her own authorship.

The author declares that the content to be published is of an academic nature and falls within the provisions defined by the Universidad Estatal de Sur de Manabí.

It is authorised to make the necessary adaptations to allow its preservation, distribution and publication in the Institutional Digital Repository of the Universidad E s t a t a t a l del Sur de Manabí.

The author, as the holder of the authorship of the work and in relation to the work, declares that the university is free from any kind of responsibility for the content of the work and that he/she assumes exclusive responsibility f o r any claims or demands from third parties.

By accepting this authorisation, t h e Universidad Estatal del Sur de Manabí is granted the exclusive right to archive and publish for consultation and citation by third parties, the work worldwide in electronic and digital format through its Institutional Digital Repository, provided that this is not done for financial gain.

Jipijapa, 4 *August* **2023**

....

....

Lorena María Loor Alvarado 1316411899

Respiratory diseases associated with biomass smoke.

Educational guide

2023

1. Overview of the guide

Title of the Guide	Respiratory diseases associated with biomass smoke.
Professional developer	**Lcda.** Lorena María Loor Alvarado
International Classification of Diseases (J00-J99)	**Chronic Obstructive Pulmonary Disease (COPD)** (J44.1) **Chronic bronchitis** (J41.0) **Pneumonia** (J67-J70)
White population	People over 18 years of age, residents of Noboa parish, diagnosed with respiratory diseases caused by biomass smoke.
Interventions and actions considered	Prevention, diagnosis, treatment, follow-up and prognosis.
Source of funding	Own
Conflicts of interest	The professional involved in the development of this guide has declared no conflict of interest in relation to the entire contents of this guide.

2. Introduction

High quality care is a priority in health care systems and is described as the provision of appropriate, efficient and effective services that generate optimal outcomes for patients, nursing is well positioned in the health care system to contribute to optimal outcomes for patients and their families (1). Building on this, the nursing care role plays a pivotal role in the care of patients suffering from respiratory diseases associated with biomass smoke. These diseases, caused primarily by prolonged exposure to the combustion of organic materials in enclosed environments, represent a major health problem worldwide, especially in rural and low-income communities.

The nursing process was initially an adapted form of problem-solving technique based on the theory used by nurses every day to help patients improve their health and to help clinicians treat patients, its main objective is to understand the health status and problems of clients who may be current or potential. It consists of a number of stages that are used to achieve the goal, the improvement of the patient's health; Assessment, Diagnosis, Planning, Implementation and Evaluation (2).

Around 3 billion individuals in various parts of the globe rely on the use of coal and biomass fuels for their heating and cooking needs. Exposure to smoke from biomass burning is linked to multiple chronic lung diseases, such as chronic obstructive pulmonary disease (COPD), asthma-COPD overlap syndrome, habitual interstitial pneumonitis, hut lung and bronchial anthracofibrosis (3).

So far, a clear causal association has been established between chronic exposure to indoor biomass fuel smoke and chronic obstructive pulmonary disease (COPD). However, the impact of acute exposures has not yet been investigated in depth. In the event that acute effects occur, there is a possibility of an increased risk of exacerbation of pre-existing lung disease(4).

Although tobacco smoke (TS) is the most common environmental risk factor and is clearly associated with COPD, exposure to biomass smoke (BS) has also been identified as a major risk factor for developing the disease, especially in non-smokers (5).

In most low- and middle-income countries, biomass cooking and heating is considered a major source of domestic and ambient air pollution, with residential biomass emissions accounting for more than 40% and 50% of the contribution to black carbon (BC)/particulate organic matter (POM) emissions respectively in South Asia, East Asia, Latin America, Europe and East Africa (6).

Addressing respiratory diseases caused by biomass smoke in rural areas is crucial to improving health outcomes, protecting vulnerable populations, promoting sustainable development, empowering communities, ensuring equity and advocating for supportive policies - a multi-faceted approach that encompasses public health, environmental conservation and social justice.

Respiratory diseases represent a major challenge for patients living in rural areas where exposure to biomass smoke is a daily reality. In these regions, many families still use fuels such as wood, charcoal or biomass for cooking and heating, resulting in regular inhalation of harmful particles, Nurses play a critical role in the care of these patients, providing personalised interventions to minimise the adverse effects of biomass smoke on their respiratory health. This guide will explore basic concepts and key nursing interventions for patients with respiratory disease in rural areas due to exposure to biomass smoke.

3. SWOT

The guideline will serve as a practical reference for clinical decision-making and contribute to quality, patient-centred nursing care and aims to provide comprehensive, evidence-based guidance for the management of patients with respiratory diseases caused by biomass smoke. By following these guidelines, nurses will be able to provide quality care, promote respiratory health and improve the well-being of affected patients.

The SWOT matrix is presented below, which aims to provide a generalised and balanced view of the situation, allowing to visualise the actions to be implemented regarding nursing interventions in patients with respiratory diseases derived from biomass smoke.

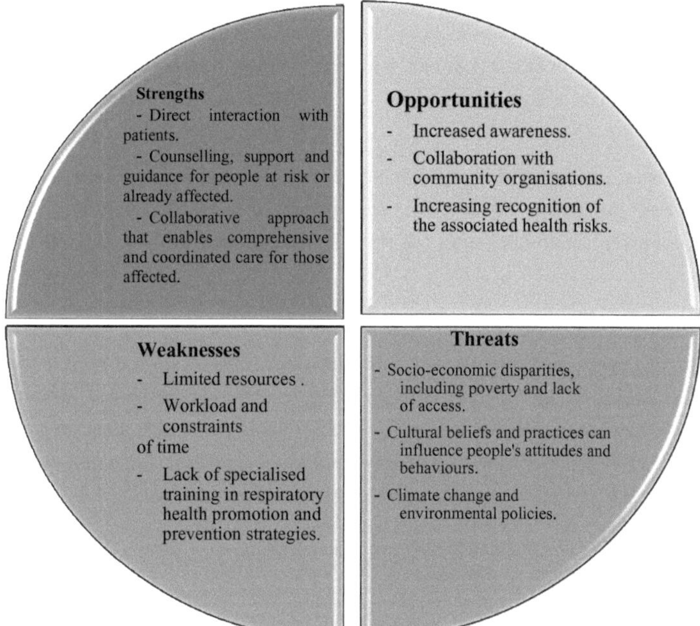

4. Benefits

The implementation of the educational guide offers a number of significant benefits to both patients and nursing professionals, such as the establishment of clear standards and protocols for the care of these patients, ensuring consistent, quality care.

It also provides guidance on the management of common respiratory symptoms such as cough, shortness of breath and sputum production, strategies to prevent complications related to respiratory diseases caused by biomass smoke, information on the disease, its management, medication, lifestyle changes and warning signs of complications, and improved health outcomes for patients.

These benefits include consistent and evidence-based care, improved management of respiratory symptoms, prevention of complications, patient and family education, care coordination and improved health outcomes, which is clinically useful for both patients and nursing professionals.

5. Targets

The goals of a nursing care guide for patients with respiratory illnesses caused by biomass smoke may vary according to the specific needs and characteristics of the patients and the community in which care is provided, it is essential to tailor goals to the individual needs of each patient and to ensure personalised, patient-centred care, and it is important to set achievable and measurable goals to assess progress and make adjustments to the care plan as needed, such as:

- Encourage patients to be active in managing their condition and promote autonomy in self-care.
- Promoting lifestyle changes that reduce exposure to biomass smoke and promote better respiratory health.
- Provide comprehensive education on the disease, triggers, warning signs, appropriate symptom management and the importance of self-care.
- Identify and address triggers, such as continued exposure to smoke, and provide strategies for prevention and management of exacerbations.

6. Respiratory diseases associated with biomass smoke.

Indoor air pollution remains a significant cause of adverse health impacts and mortality, especially in developing countries. In these countries, around 50% of households and 90% of rural households use biofuels for cooking, which is the main source of indoor air pollution. Recent estimates indicate that between 1.5 and 2 million people die annually due to indoor air pollution, and of these, approximately 1 million are children under 5 years of age suffering from acute respiratory infections (7).

The most common respiratory diseases caused by biomass smoke include:

6.1. Chronic Obstructive Pulmonary Disease (COPD)

Chronic obstructive pulmonary disease (COPD) is a common and potentially life-threatening respiratory condition that affects millions of people worldwide. It is characterised by a chronic inflammatory response in the airways, often triggered by exposure to tobacco smoke(8).

The Spanish Society of Pneumology and Thoracic Surgery (SEPAR) indicates that chronic obstructive pulmonary disease (COPD) is a chronic respiratory disease caused by the inhalation of a toxic substance, usually tobacco. It causes airflow obstruction and difficulty in emptying air from the lungs. This damage causes the walls of the alveoli to be destroyed, the bronchi to thicken and the lungs to produce more mucus than normal, causing the airways to become obstructed. Spirometry is a simple, painless test that takes 10 minutes. It aids in the diagnosis, treatment and monitoring of COPD(9).

Relative to unexposed individuals, those exposed to biomass smoke have an odds ratio of 2.44 (95 % CI, 1.9-3.33) for developing COPD, while among women over 30 years of age who performed household chores predominantly in rural areas, the relative risk of COPD was estimated at 3.2 (95 % CI, 2.3-4.8) [41] or 2.14 (95 % CI, 1.78-2.58) (10).

6.1.1. Prevention

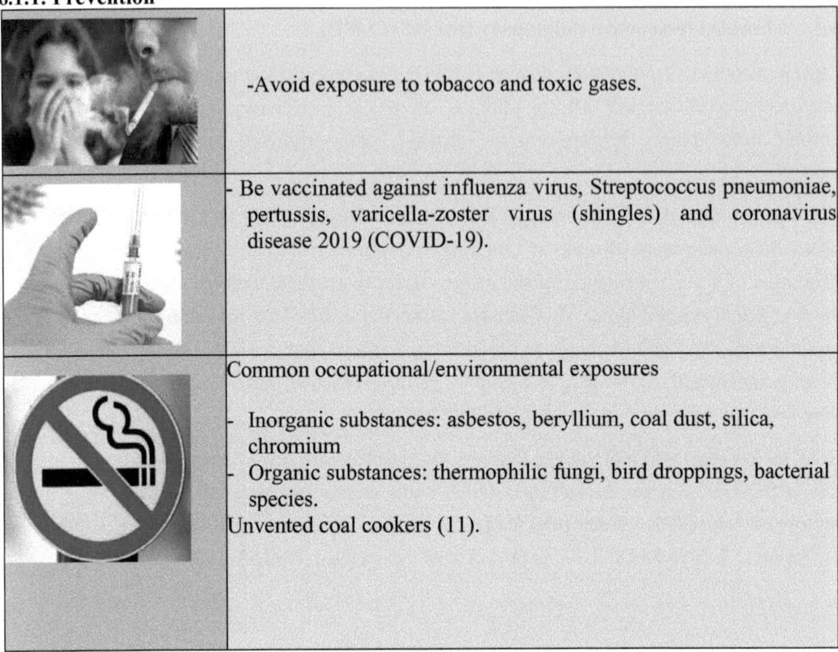

	-Avoid exposure to tobacco and toxic gases.
	- Be vaccinated against influenza virus, Streptococcus pneumoniae, pertussis, varicella-zoster virus (shingles) and coronavirus disease 2019 (COVID-19).
	Common occupational/environmental exposures - Inorganic substances: asbestos, beryllium, coal dust, silica, chromium - Organic substances: thermophilic fungi, bird droppings, bacterial species. Unvented coal cookers (11).

6.1.2. Diagnostic

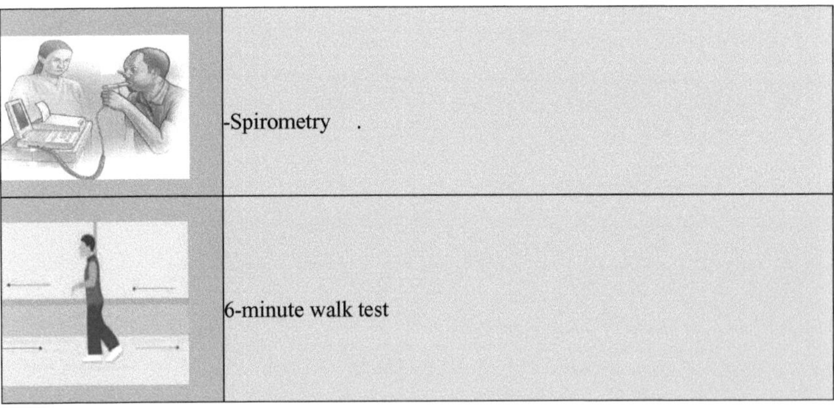

	-Spirometry .
	6-minute walk test

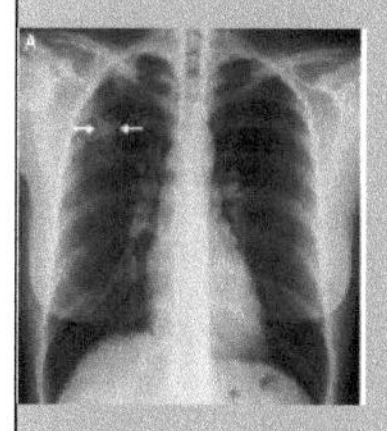	Chest X-ray and computed tomography (CT) (12).

6.1.3. Treatment

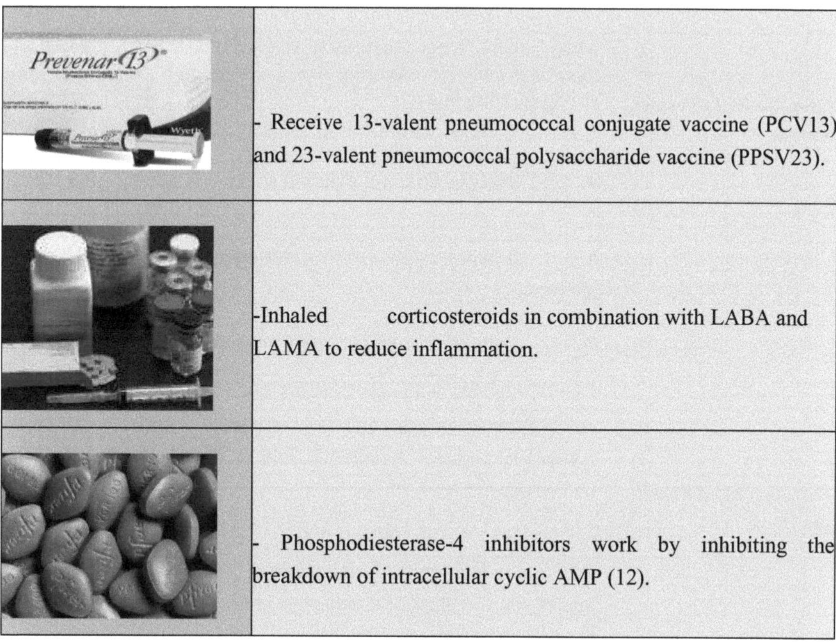

	- Receive 13-valent pneumococcal conjugate vaccine (PCV13) and 23-valent pneumococcal polysaccharide vaccine (PPSV23).
	-Inhaled corticosteroids in combination with LABA and LAMA to reduce inflammation.
	- Phosphodiesterase-4 inhibitors work by inhibiting the breakdown of intracellular cyclic AMP (12).

6.1.4. Monitoring

-Regular assessment of respiratory symptoms, such as cough, dyspnoea and sputum production, using standardised assessment scales.
-Patient education on COPD and its management.
-Providing support to the patient in complying with the prescribed treatment.

-Pulmonary function tests, such as spirometry, to assess the patient's respiratory capacity (12).

6.1.5. Living with the disease

Maintain an active life Nutrition and diet	Malnutrition is common, especially in severe patients, and can affect up to 50% of cases. Malnutrition worsens lung function, quality of life and muscle strength, and in turn increases the likelihood of an exacerbation of the disease due to impaired immune response (defences) (13).
Exercise and physical activity	Many patients reduce their usual level of physical activity to avoid dyspnoea and, for example, stop walking and spend more time sitting or lying down: • It improves the use of oxygen needed and used by your body. • Improve your muscles and joints.
	• It improves your heart, cardiovascular system and blood pressure. • It improves COPD symptoms, especially dyspnoea (13).
Getting a good night's sleep	COPD, together with other factors such as obesity, smoking and alcohol consumption, may contribute to a disorder called Sleep Apnoea-Hypopnoea Syndrome, which should be assessed and treated appropriately (13).
Overcoming anxiety/depression	When you feel stressed and anxious, you breathe faster, which makes you feel short of breath. The greater the shortness of breath, the greater the anxiety. People with COPD who are depressed are at increased risk of flare-ups and are more likely to go to hospital. Depression saps their energy and motivation (13).
Travel and leisure	• Think about the climate of the place you want to visit (avoid extreme temperatures: neither too hot nor too cold), the terrain you will have to move around (flat and sea level places are more affordable), the means of transport to the destination. • Discuss the trip with your doctor, who will tell you whether you are fit to travel (13).

6.2. Chronic bronchitis

persistent cough and sputum production is commonly referred to as one of the most common and most reported conditions worldwide, with chronic bronchitis characterised by a chronic increase in mucoid bronchial secretions (10).

Chronic bronchitis is associated with inflammation within the central airways (defined as greater than 4 mm internal diameter), transformation into mucus-producing glands and bronchial wall thickening associated with extracellular matrix deposition. While most smokers will develop chronic bronchitis during their lifetime, the presence of chronic bronchitis alone does not predict the development or progression of airflow limitation (14).

Chronic bronchitis is thought to be caused by overproduction and hypersecretion of mucus by goblet cells, the epithelial cells lining the airways that respond to toxic and infectious stimuli by releasing inflammatory mediators such as interleukin-8, colony-stimulating factor and other proinflammatory cytokines, colony-stimulating factor and other pro-inflammatory cytokines, and there is also an associated decrease in the release of regulatory substances such as angiotensin-converting enzyme and neutral endopeptidase (15).

6.2.1. Prevention

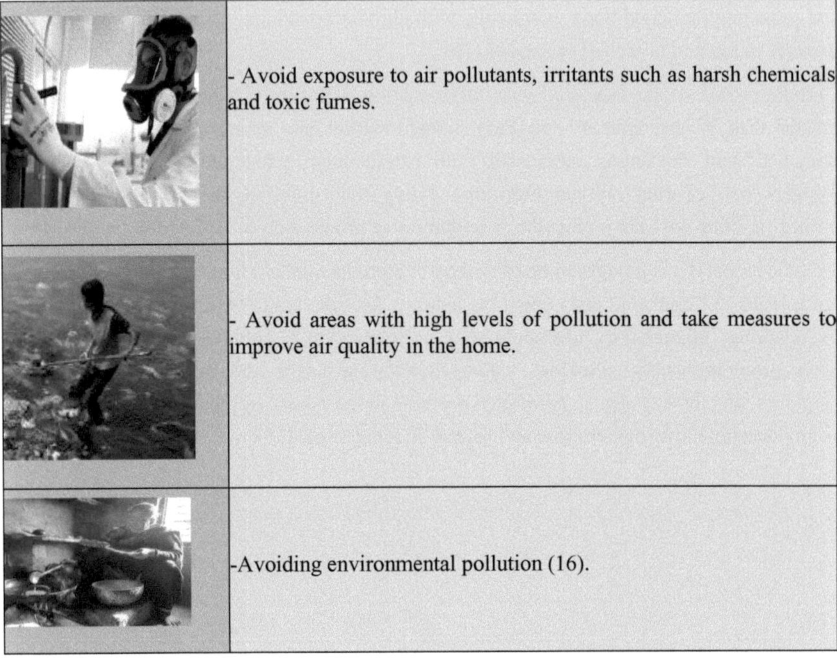

- Avoid exposure to air pollutants, irritants such as harsh chemicals and toxic fumes.

- Avoid areas with high levels of pollution and take measures to improve air quality in the home.

-Avoiding environmental pollution (16).

6.2.2. Diagnostic

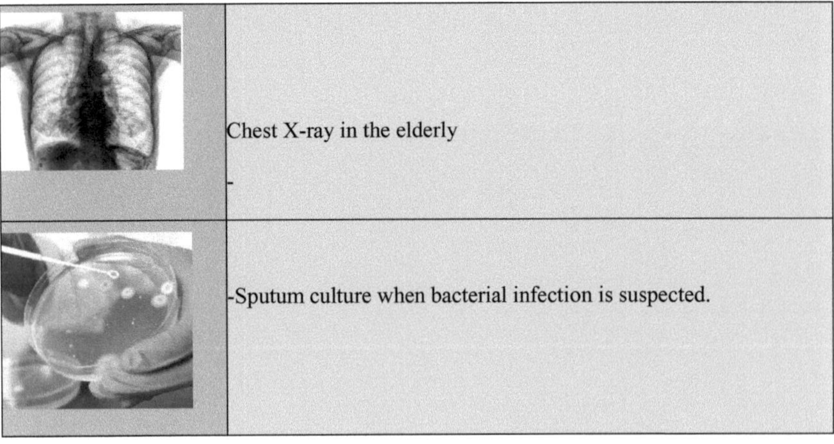

Chest X-ray in the elderly

-

-Sputum culture when bacterial infection is suspected.

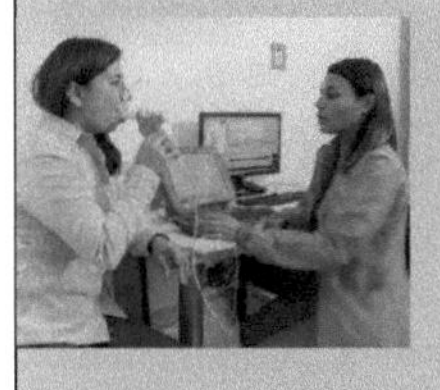	-Oxygen saturation and pulmonary function test (16).

6.2.3. Treatment

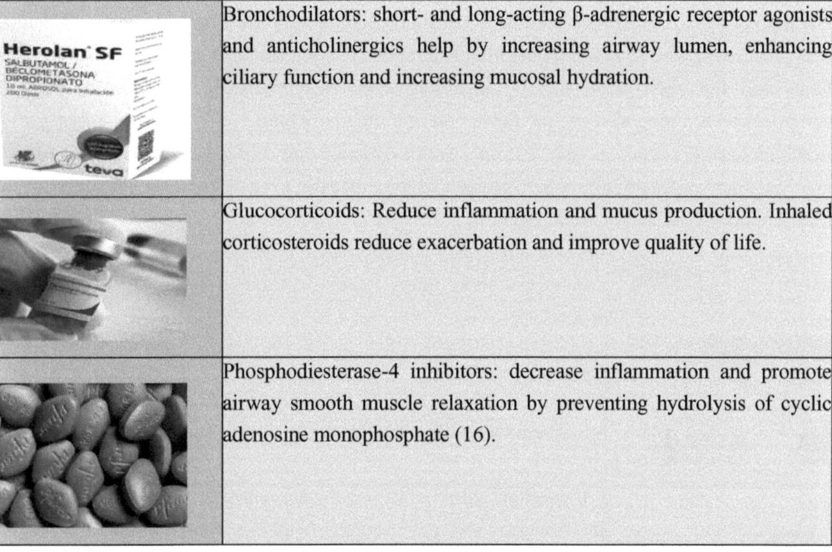

Herolan SF SALBUTAMOL / BECLOMETASONA DIPROPIONATO teva	Bronchodilators: short- and long-acting β-adrenergic receptor agonists and anticholinergics help by increasing airway lumen, enhancing ciliary function and increasing mucosal hydration.
	Glucocorticoids: Reduce inflammation and mucus production. Inhaled corticosteroids reduce exacerbation and improve quality of life.
	Phosphodiesterase-4 inhibitors: decrease inflammation and promote airway smooth muscle relaxation by preventing hydrolysis of cyclic adenosine monophosphate (16).

6.2.4. Monitoring

- Support patient compliance with prescribed treatment, ensuring that they understand how and when to take medicines, how to use inhalation devices correctly and what to do if they miss a dose.
-Adopt a healthy lifestyle that reduces risk factors and improves respiratory health.

Nursing follow-up in patients with chronic bronchitis is essential to provide comprehensive care and improve the patient's quality of life.

6.3. Pneumonia

Pneumonia is a disease that affects the tissues of the lung. When a person contracts pneumonia, the small air sacs in the lungs, called alveoli, fill with microorganisms, fluid and inflammatory cells, preventing the lungs from functioning properly. The diagnosis of pneumonia is based on symptoms and signs of an acute lower respiratory tract infection, and can be confirmed by a chest x-ray showing a new shadow that is not due to any other cause, such as pulmonary oedema or infarction (17).

Pneumonia can cause inflammation of the lining that covers the lungs (pulmonary pleura), which causes severe pain when coughing or breathing. Fluid can also accumulate between the lungs and the chest wall, making breathing even more difficult, and another possible complication is a lung abscess, the formation of a lung lung lung lung abscess . Epidemiological studies in Asia, Europe, South America and Africa have consistently shown links between exposure to biomass smoke and lung disease, even after taking into account the most important risk factor, smoking (18).

6.3.1. Prevention

	-Limit contact with cigarette smoke or stop smoking.
	- Implement community-level interventions, such as clean energy programmes and environmental policies that promote the use of cleaner fuels.
	- Encourage the use of cleaner fuels, such as liquefied petroleum gas (LPG), electricity or clean-burning cookers (19).

6.3.2. Diagnosis

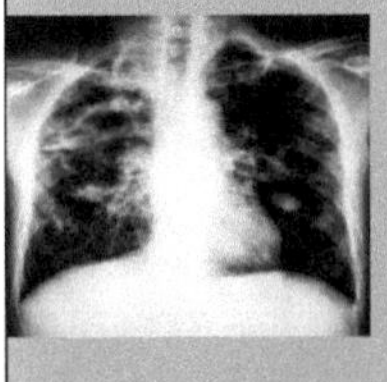

Radiological evaluation

- A demonstrable chest radiographic infiltrate is required and is considered the best method (with supporting clinical findings) for the diagnosis of pneumonia.

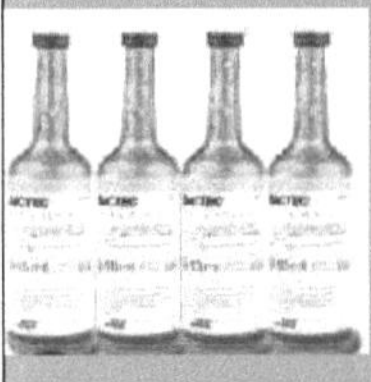

Laboratory evaluation

- Blood culture, sputum culture and microscopy, routine blood counts and lymphocyte counts. For certain pathogens, special tests such as urinary antigen testing, bronchial aspirate or induced sputum may be used.

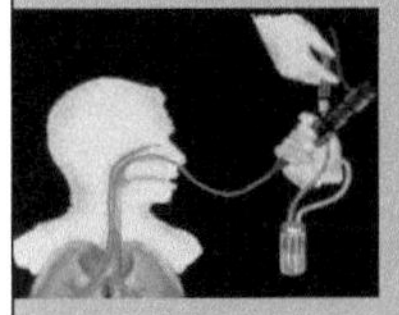

- Invasive sampling techniques such as mini bronchoalveolar lavage (BAL) or bronchoscopic BAL or even protected sample brush (PSB) to identify causative organisms (19).

6.3.3. Treatment

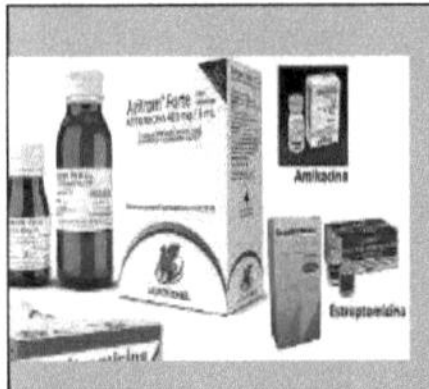

A score of 0 to 1: Outpatient management. These patients are treated empirically with Fluoroquinolones or Beta-lactams + Macrolides if they have adverse comorbidities and with Macrolides or Doxycycline if they do not have comorbidities.

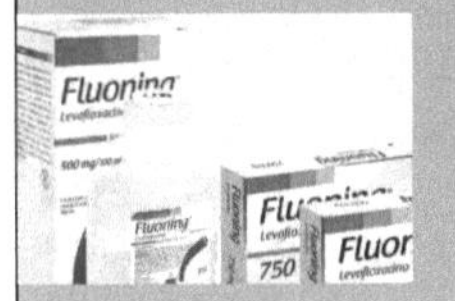

A score of 2 to 3 indicates admission and management in a general medicine ward. The first line of treatment is the choice between fluoroquinolones or macrolides plus beta-lactams.

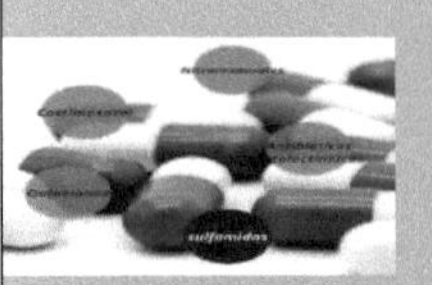	A score of 4 or more warrants management in an ICU. The empiric regimen, in this case, is a choice between a combination of a beta-lactam plus fluoroquinolones or beta-lactams plus macrolides (19).

6.3.4. Monitoring

-Monitor the patient's oxygen saturation using a pulse oximeter and adjust oxygen administration as necessary.
- Encourage patients to mobilise and perform deep breathing exercises and assisted coughing to help clear secretions from the lungs.
-Watch for any signs of complications, such as respiratory failure, pleural effusion or sepsis (19).

6.4. Types of biomass used in rural areas.

The most commonly used types of biomass in rural areas are fuelwood, agricultural and forestry residues, dung and liquid biofuels such as biodiesel.

Wood: Wood and charcoal are the most popular and widely used fuel types due to their ease and low cost of production, especially in developing countries, in contrast, in most developing countries where the study of the "wood fuel problem" has been concentrated, woody biomass is used in both rural and urban areas in low efficiency cooking cookers (20).

According to the World Health Organisation (WHO), smoke-induced diseases are responsible for the deaths of 4.3 million people each year (more deaths than those caused by malaria or tuberculosis), making them one of the most lethal environmental health hazards worldwide(21).

Young children are particularly vulnerable for two reasons: first, they are usually with their mothers during the cooking process and therefore inhale large amounts of emitted particles (21).

Secondly, compared to adults, the still growing bodies of young children are more susceptible to ARI, leading to a high mortality rate in this age group (22).

Smoke from agricultural and forest residues: Like smoke from forest fires, smoke from agricultural burning can have harmful effects on public health. To protect public health, Northwest smoke control agencies regulate agricultural burning by deciding how much, if any, field burning can occur on a given day (23).

Burning crop residues contributes to poor air quality and imposes a health burden in India. Despite government bans and other interventions, the practice is still widespread (24).

Manure: Burning this material in open fires and cookers results in high concentrations of particulate matter (PM), carbon monoxide, nitrogen dioxide, as well as volatile and semi-volatile organic species in the indoor environment, manure is often burned many times a day for heating and cooking, humans on at least five continents collect manure from a variety of different herd animals (25).

Biodiesel: The most widespread alternative to mineral diesel is biodiesel, biodiesel is a generic term used to describe fuel that can be made from a wide variety of vegetable or animal oils through a process known as transesterification, globally, the use of solid fuels in homes is the leading cause of indoor air pollution, exposure to by-products resulting from the combustion of bio-based fuels, especially wood smoke, has been associated with various respiratory disorders, as well as increased mortality and disease burden (26).

6.5. Extramural or community care provided mainly by first-level operational facilities:

The objective is health care through measures aimed at identifying and controlling risks at the individual, family, community and environmental levels, implementing strategies and actions for prevention, health promotion, health education, strengthening citizen participation and intersectoral coordination to act on the determinants of health and contribute to integrated development at the local level.

It is mainly carried out by the Integrated Care Teams at the first level of care, who carry it out:

a) Community organisation activities involving social actors in the coverage area to work on the population's priority problems.

b) Timely identification of risks and/or harm to individuals, families and the community and implementation of care plans.

c) Systematic health promotion activities at individual, family and community level.

d) Attention to priority populations and remote communities.

e) Identify sentinel events for the implementation of timely epidemiological measures.

6.5.1. Home-based work

Home care. Medical and/or nursing care for people who, due to illness, disability, emergency or terminal illness, [illegible]care and are unable to travel to the unit.

In addition, the integrated health team will be obliged to monitor and evaluate these people.

Timely identification of risks and/or damage to individuals, families, the community and the environment and implementation of care plans: Home visits for diagnosis and monitoring of families at risk through the application of the family record and preparation of the intervention plan.

These actions will be developed with scheduled home visits, it is not necessary for all the staff of the teams to go out to carry out this activity.

- Early detection and comprehensive care of health problems: mental, biological, impairments and disabilities such as physical, motor, intellectual, hearing, visual; and social in priority groups,23 elaboration, implementation, registration and evaluation of interventions.
- Identification, care and support of palliative care for terminally ill persons and the family.
- Dynamic, organised and continuous assessment of the state of health of people in their family and/or social environment, with the aim of influencing its improvement through the planning and development of actions that contribute to it.
- Identification of environmental risks and occupational groups at risk, elaboration and implementation, registration and evaluation of intervention plans with cross-sectoral intervention (27).

6.6. Intervention actions

1. Assessment of respiratory function, including pulmonary auscultation and measurement of vital signs.
2. Education on the risks associated with exposure to biomass smoke and the importance of reducing exposure.
3. Teaching breathing techniques and lung expansion exercises to improve respiratory function.
4. Monitoring of oxygen saturation and administration of supplemental oxygen if necessary.
5. Administration of bronchodilator and anti-inflammatory drugs according to medical prescription.
6. Encouragement of physical activity and regular exercise to strengthen respiratory muscles.
7. Education on the importance of maintaining a smoke-free environment and avoiding the use of biomass fuels.
8. Promotion of adequate ventilation in dwellings and education on methods to improve ventilation.
9. Teaching effective coughing techniques to help clear lung secretions.
10. Encouraging the adoption of safer cooking practices, such as the use of improved cookers or adequate ventilation systems.

11. Education on the importance of maintaining good personal hygiene to prevent respiratory infections.

12. Collaboration with local authorities and community organisations to promote the use of cleaner technologies.

13. Regular assessment and monitoring of respiratory symptoms to adjust the care plan as needed.

14. Emotional support and education on stress management, as stress can worsen respiratory symptoms.

15. Encouraging participation in community education programmes on respiratory health and disease prevention.

16. Assessment and management of respiratory complications, such as exacerbations of chronic diseases.

17. Advice on the use of air purifiers or filters in rural areas to reduce exposure to harmful particles.

18. Nutritional support to maintain a healthy diet and strengthen the immune system.

19. Referral and coordination of specialised health services when necessary, taking into account resource constraints in rural areas.

20. Promoting adherence to medical treatment and long-term follow-up to monitor disease progression and prevent complications.

7. References

1. Smolowitz J, Speakman E, Wojnar D, Whelan EM, Ulrich S, Hayes C, et al. Role of the registered nurse in primary health care: meeting health care needs in the 21st century. Nurs Outlook [Internet]. 2015 Mar 1 [cited 2023 Jun 15];63(2):130-6. Available from: https://pubmed.ncbi.nlm.nih.gov/25261382/

2. Ebisa Z, Abebe D, Meseret R, Eshetu E C, Guta kune. Implementation of Nursing Process and Its' Associated Factors among Nurses' Working at Public Hospitals of Central Ethiopian, 2020; Institutional Based Cross-sectional Study. Journal of Nursing and Practice. 2022 Jul 23;5(3):473-9.

3. Assad NA, Kapoor V, Sood A. Biomass smoke exposure and chronic lung disease. Curr Opin Pulm Med [Internet]. 2016 Mar 1 [cited 2023 May 23];22(2):150-7. Available from: https://pubmed.ncbi.nlm.nih.gov/26814722/

4. Kurmi OP, Gaihre S, Semple S, Ayres JG. Acute exposure to biomass smoke causes oxygen desaturation in adult women. Thorax [Internet]. [cited 2023 May 23];66(8):724-

5. Available from: https://thorax.bmj.com/content/66/8/724

5. Olloquequi J, Rafael Silva O. Biomass smoke as a risk factor for chronic obstructive pulmonary disease: Effects on innate immunity. Innate Immun [Internet]. 2016 Jul 1 [cited 2023 May 23];22(5):373-81. Available from: https://journals.sagepub.com/doi/10.1177/1753425916650272

6. Adhikari S, Mahapatra PS, Pokheral CP, Puppala SP. Cookstove Smoke Impact on Ambient Air Quality and Probable Consequences for Human Health in Rural Locations of Southern Nepal. International Journal of Environmental Research and Public Health 2020, Vol 17, Page 550 [Internet]. 2020 Jan 15 [cited 2023 May 23];17(2):550. Available from: https://www.mdpi.com/1660-4601/17/2/550/htm

7. Alvis-Guzman N, De la Hoz-Restrepo F, Montes-Farah J, Paternina-Caicedo A. Effect of biomass smoke on chronic obstructive pulmonary disease in rural localities of Colombia. Revista de Salud Pública [Internet]. [cited 2023 May 23];15(4):638-50. Available from: http://www.scielo.org.co/scielo.php?script=sci_arttext&pid=S0124-00642013000400009&lng=en&nrm=iso&tlng=en

8. Szalontai K, Gémes N, Furák J, Varga T, Neuperger P, Balog J, et al. Chronic Obstructive Pulmonary Disease: Epidemiology, Biomarkers, and Paving the Way to Lung Cancer. J Clin Med [Internet]. 2021 Jul 1 [cited 2023 May 23];10(13):2889. Available from: /pmc/articles/PMC8268950/

9. Spanish Society of Pneumology and Thoracic Surgery. COPD [Internet]. 2020 [cited 2023 Jul 30]. Available from: https://www.separ.es/node/975

10. Apte K, Salvi S, Hoek G, Sunyer J. Household air pollution and its effects on health. F1000Research 2016 5:2593 [Internet]. 2016 Oct 28 [cited 2023 May 23];5:2593. Available

from: https://f1000research.com/articles/5-2593

11. Respiratory EC. Advances In Respiratory Care | Prevention. [cited 2023 Jun 16]; Available from: https://www.avancesenrespiratorio.com/prevencion_epoc

12. Zatloukal J, Brat K, Neumannova K, Volakova E, Hejduk K, Kocova E, et al. Chronic obstructive pulmonary disease - diagnosis and management of stable disease; a personalized approach to care, using the treatable traits concept based on clinical phenotypes. Position paper of the czech pneumological and phthisiological society. Biomedical Papers. 2020 Dec 1;164(4):325-56.

13. SEPAR. "LIVING WITH COPD: A NEW GUIDE FOR PATIENTS AND CAREGIVERS FROM RESPIRA PUBLISHERS | separ [Internet]. 2016 [cited 2023 Jul 30]. Available from: https://www.separ.es/node/557

14. Hackett TL, Polverino F, Kheradmand F. Chronic Obstructive Pulmonary Disease and Emphysema. Clinical Immunology: Principles and Practice, Sixth Edition. 2023 Jan 1;936-42.

15. Jetmalani K, Thamrin C, Farah CS, Bertolin A, Chapman DG, Berend N, et al. Peripheral airway dysfunction and relationship with symptoms in smokers with preserved spirometry. Respirology [Internet]. 2018 May 1 [cited 2023 May 26];23(5):512-8. Available from: https://onlinelibrary.wiley.com/doi/full/10.1111/resp.13215

16. Widysanto A, Mathew G. Chronic Bronchitis. Adjuvant Medical Care [Internet]. 2022 Nov 28 [cited 2023 Jun 16];39-41. Available from: https://www.ncbi.nlm.nih.gov/books/NBK482437/

17. (NICE) NI for H and CE. Pneumonia in adults: diagnosis and management. 2022 Jul 7 [cited 2023 May 26]; Available from: https://www.ncbi.nlm.nih.gov/books/NBK552669/

18. KC R, Shukla SD, Gautam SS, Hansbro PM, O'Toole RF. The role of environmental exposure to non-cigarette smoke in lung disease. Clin Transl Med [Internet]. 2018 Dec [cited 2023 May 26];7(1):39. Available from: /pmc/articles/PMC6279673/

19. Jain V, Vashisht R, Yilmaz G, Bhardwaj A. Pneumonia Pathology. StatPearls [Internet]. 2022 Aug 1 [cited 2023 Jun 16]; Available from: https://www.ncbi.nlm.nih.gov/books/NBK526116/

20. Reyes R, Nelson H, Zerriffi H. Firewood: Cause or consequence? Underlying drivers of firewood production in the South of Chile. Energy for Sustainable Development. 2018 Feb 1;42:97-108.

21. Diekman ST, Pope D, Falk H, Ballesteros MF, Dherani M, Johnson NG, et al. WHO Indoor Air Quality Guidelines: Household Fuel Combustion. [cited 2023 May 27]; Available from: http://www.who.int/indoorair/guidelines/hhfc

22. Barnes BR. Behavioural Change, Indoor Air Pollution and Child Respiratory Health in Developing Countries: A Review. International Journal of Environmental Research and Public Health 2014, Vol 11, Pages 4607-4618 [Internet]. 2014 Apr 25 [cited 2023 May 27];11(5):4607-18. Available from: https://www.mdpi.com/1660-4601/11/5/4607/htm

23. Elleman R. Washington State University. 2015 [cited 2023 May 28]. Agricultural Smoke

| Missoula Fire Sciences Laboratory. Available from: https://www.firelab.org/project/agricultural-smoke

24. Lan R, Eastham SD, Liu T, Norford LK, Barrett SRH. Air quality impacts of crop residue burning in India and mitigation alternatives. Nature Communications 2022 13:1 [Internet]. 2022 Nov 14 [cited 2023 May 28];13(1):1-13. Available from: https://www.nature.com/articles/s41467-022-34093-z

25. Spengler RN. Dung burning in the archaeobotanical record of West Asia: where are we now? Veg Hist Archaeobot [Internet]. 2019 May 15 [cited 2023 May 28];28(3):215-27. Available from: https://link.springer.com/article/10.1007/s00334-018-0669-8

26. Larcombe AN, Kicic A, Mullins BJ, Knothe G. Biodiesel exhaust: The need for a systematic approach to health effects research. Respirology [Internet]. 2015 Oct 1 [cited 2023 May 28];20(7):1034-45. Available from: https://onlinelibrary.wiley.com/doi/full/10.1111/resp.12587

27. MSP ECUADOR. Manual del Modelo de Atención Integral de Salud - MAIS [Internet]. Ecuador; 2018 [cited2023Jun12]. 210p. Available from: https://www.hgdc.gob.ec/images/DocumentosInstitucionales/Manual_MAIS-MSP12.12.12.pdf

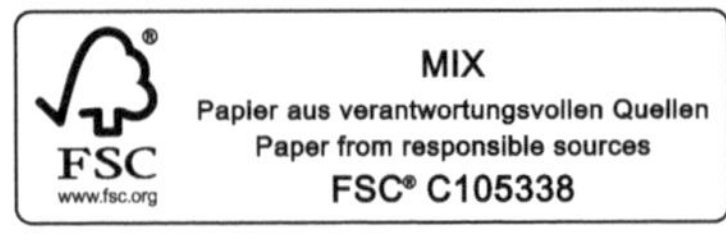

Printed by Books on Demand GmbH, Norderstedt / Germany